Comprehensive Intervention for Children with Developmental Delays

Program Manual and Checklists

Comprehensive Intervention for Children with Developmental Delays

Program Manual and Checklists

Prathibha Karanth, PhD
Priya James, MS, CCC-SLP

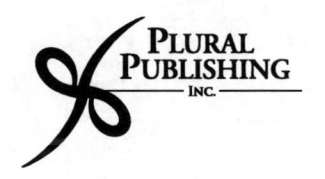

Plural Publishing, Inc.

Plural Publishing, Inc.

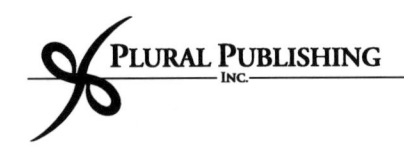

5521 Ruffin Road
San Diego, CA 92123

e-mail: info@pluralpublishing.com
Website: http://www.pluralpublishing.com

Copyright © 2017 by Plural Publishing, Inc.

Typeset in 11/13 Palatino by Flanagan's Publishing Services, Inc.
Printed in the United States of America by McNaughton & Gunn, Inc.

All rights, including that of translation, reserved. No part of this publication may be reproduced, stored in a retrieval system, or transmitted in any form or by any means, electronic, mechanical, recording, or otherwise, including photocopying, recording, taping, Web distribution, or information storage and retrieval systems without the prior written consent of the publisher.

For permission to use material from this text, contact us by
Telephone: (866) 758-7251
Fax: (888) 758-7255
e-mail: permissions@pluralpublishing.com

Every attempt has been made to contact the copyright holders for material originally printed in another source. If any have been inadvertently overlooked, the publishers will gladly make the necessary arrangements at the first opportunity.

Library of Congress Cataloging-in-Publication Data

Names: Karanth, Prathibha, author. | James, Priya, author.
Title: Comprehensive intervention for children with developmental delays : program manual and checklists / Prathibha Karanth, Priya James.
Description: San Diego, CA : Plural Publishing, [2017] | Includes bibliographical references.
Identifiers: LCCN 2017010594 | ISBN 9781597569712 (alk. paper) | ISBN 1597569712 (alk. paper)
Subjects: | MESH: Neurodevelopmental Disorders--therapy | Child, Preschool | Speech-Language Pathology—methods | Early Intervention (Education)—methods
Classification: LCC RJ496.S7 | NLM WS 350.6 | DDC 618.92/855—dc23
LC record available at https://lccn.loc.gov/2017010594

Contents

Acknowledgments   *vii*
Project Team   *viii*

SECTION 1   **Introduction**   1

SECTION 2   **Background**   3

SECTION 3   **Communication DEALL**   9
    3.1 The Program   9
        3.1.1 Theoretical Framework   9
        3.1.2 The Com DEALL Intervention Model   13
        3.1.3 The Team   14
        3.1.4 Flow of the Program   14
        3.1.5 Time Frame   15
        3.1.6 Assessment   16
        3.1.7 Intervention   16
    3.2 Com DEALL Manuals   17

SECTION 4   **The Communication DEALL Developmental Checklists**   19
    4.1 Executive Summary   19
        4.1.1 Background   19
        4.1.2 Statistical Background   20
        4.1.3 Directions for Use   24
        4.1.4 Scoring   25
        4.1.5 Interpretation   28
    4.2 Checklists   29
        4.2.1 Gross Motor Skills   29
        4.2.2 Fine Motor Skills   31
        4.2.3 Activities of Daily Living   33
        4.2.4 Receptive Language   35
        4.2.5 Expressive Language   37
        4.2.6 Cognitive Skills   39
        4.2.7 Social Skills   41
        4.2.8 Emotional Skills   43
    4.3 Alternative and Augmentative Communication   45

SECTION 5   **The Profiles**   47
    5.1 Normal Development   48
    5.2 Normal Development   49

5.3	Autism Spectrum Disorder	50
5.4	ASD	51
5.5	Sensory Processing Disorder with Apraxia	52
5.6	Specific Language Impairment	53
5.7	Developmental Delay	54
5.8	Cerebral Palsy	55
5.9	Profile 9—Monitoring Progress	56
5.10	Profile 10—Monitoring Progress	57

SECTION 6 Research on the Communication DEALL Program 59

6.1 Efficacy Study 59
6.2 Long-Term Outcome 60
6.3 Prerequisite Learning Skills 60
6.4 Oral Motor/Motor Issues 61

SECTION 7 Update on the Com DEALL Program 63

7.1 Com DEALL Units 63
    7.1.1 Scaling Up the Com DEALL Model 63
    7.1.2 Setting Up of a Com DEALL Unit 63
7.2 New Clinical Programs 64
    7.2.1 The Pre DEALL Program 64
    7.2.2 FMIP: Family Mediated Intervention (Home Training) Programs 64

References 65
Appendix. CDDC Score Sheets 67

Acknowledgments

The Communication Developmental Eclectic Approach to Language Learning (DEALL) program was designed and developed by the first author as an Early Intervention program for children with Autism Spectrum Disorders in Bengaluru, India, in 2000. The documentation of the program took place from 2005 to 2010 and it continues to grow in many ways. There have been several individuals who have contributed to the growth of the program, and it is not possible to acknowledge each of them independently here. The first author would like to acknowledge the contribution of the Tata Trust, Mumbai, India, for their grant support from 2005 to date, which enabled the documentation and scaling up of the project. Key persons whose commitment contributed significantly to the program over the years are Deepa Bhat Nair, Nirupama Srikanth, Tanushree Saxena-Chandok and Ujwala Aluri. The team members who worked on the individual manuals are acknowledged in the respective manuals. All of the staff who worked on the Communication DEALL program since 2000 to date, the many functionaries of the Tata Trust who interacted with us on this project from time to time, and many other well-wishers have enriched these manuals. For this international edition, the first author is grateful to her American collaborators, Celeste Roseberry-McKibbin for her significant contribution to the nine intervention manuals, and Priya James for being instrumental in bringing these manuals to the international forum. With much gratitude, we acknowledge: Sneha Susan Jacob and Vidya Ramesh, who helped us in building CDDC profiles of children with various disabilities for this international edition; Linda Pippert and Katie Vorreiter for editing the Com DEALL developmental checklist for the western population; and Brian Ou Yang, our artist, who did an amazing job in illustrating more than one hundred images. We also want to thank Angie Singh, Valerie Johns, Kalie Koscielak, Linda Shapiro and Jessica Bristow of Plural Publishing for their patience and support and all the staff involved in this project at Plural Publishing.

Prathibha Karanth would like to acknowledge Ullas, Krithi, and Avinash for their support and Keya and Ayla for the joy they bring to everything.

Priya James would like to acknowledge, "My husband Saiju and my son Bharat for their constant support and love. My parents, without their sacrifice I wouldn't have been able to finish this project and my uncle Dr. A D Antony whose passion has always been an inspiration."

Project Team

Prathibha Karanth Principal Investigator (Sep 2007 to Dec 2010)		
Nirupama Srikanth Coordinator (Sep 2007 to Dec 2010)		**Antony Roche** Illustrator (Oct 2007 to Dec 2010)
Speech Language Pathologists	**Occupational Therapists**	**Developmental Educators**
Tanushree Saxena-Chandbok (Sep 07 to Nov 10)	Animesh Manjhi (Nov 09 to Nov 10)	Lekshmi Priya (Sep 07 to Nov 10)
Poornima Ram-Kiran (Oct 07 to Feb 09)	Priscilla Fredrick (June 09 to Jan 10)	Lakshmi M. (Sep 07 to Aug 09)
Archana S (Aug 09 to Oct 10)	Sherry Bhatra (July 08 to Dec 08)	Gifty Paulson (Nov 09 to Nov 10)
Susan Chacko Libu (July 09 to June 10)	Shruti Bhide (Feb 08 to April 08)	
Usha Nayar Counselor (June 08 to Nov 10)		Lathina Lawrance Social Worker (Aug 09 to Sep 10)

Introduction

The Communication Developmental Eclectic Approach to Language Learning (DEALL) was formally initiated in Bangalore, India, in November 2000. However, the clinical insights that influenced the program date back to the 1970s and the decades that followed, during which I was increasingly involved with children with developmental language disorders, who while not being labeled with autism (ASD), nevertheless showed signs of autism and were later covered by the term 'pervasive developmental disorders.' It was, however, my decade-long work with Tito Rajarishi Mukhophadhyay during the 1990s (Mukhopadhyay, 2000), and the steep increase in the number of families with children with ASD that sought our help, coupled with the total lack of concerted services for these children, even in metropolitan cities like Bangalore, that eventually led to the setting up of the Communication DEALL program.

Communication DEALL is an early intervention program for children with communication disorders such as Specific Language Impairment (SLI), Developmental Verbal Dyspraxia (DVD), Pervasive Developmental Disorder (PDD), and Autism Spectrum Disorder (ASD). The aim of this program is the integration of these children into regular schools, with intensive preschool intervention, to the extent possible. It provides multidisciplinary intervention to small groups of 12 children, in the age range of 0 to 6 years, three hours per weekday, from a minimum of one year of intervention to a maximum of three years of intervention, with the goal of integrating them into regular school by the school entry age of 6 years.

Since its initiation, the program has been vetted and continuously fine-tuned over the last decade and a half. In the pages that follow we have described how, when, and why the program was started. The scientific framework of the program has been given. Development and administration of assessment procedures are described. This is followed by illustration of individual profiles of children with Autism Spectrum Disorders and other communication disorders. These profiles serve as the basis for initiating and monitoring intervention as specified in the intervention manuals.

Background

The clinical experiences that I had gained over several years, while working with adult patients with neurogenic communication disorders at the National Institute of Mental Health and Neurosciences (NIMHANS), in Bangalore, and the research and teaching experiences that followed in the same area, while at the All India Institute of Speech & Hearing (AIISH), Mysore, stood me in good stead during my decade-long involvement with Tito Rajrishi Mukhopdhyay, a gifted child with autism who was later to become 'the poster boy' of Autism in the United States.

Tito first came to AIISH in Mysore, India, with a referral for a hearing assessment from the Department of Psychiatry of Christian Medical College (CMC), Vellore, India, in April 1993. He was then 3 years, 8 months old and was being investigated at CMC for autism. The audiological evaluation at AIISH suggested that his hearing was within normal limits. The psychologist's report, while listing several characteristic signs of autism, recommended further observation to confirm the diagnosis. What drew our attention to Tito was the observation that while he hardly spoke, with assistance from his mother, he spelled out complex words and phrases in English. The method used was to direct his mother's pointed finger at the letters on an alphabet board—what to us appeared as a version of the facilitated communication that had resulted in heated debate in the United States not too long ago. His mother carried a little notebook that documented the snippets of conversation and poetry that had reportedly emerged from this nonverbal, seemingly autistic child of 4 years, with much of the content well above the capabilities of his peers. However, given the particular mode of communication used, there was understandably considerable skepticism whether what was being spelled out was indeed his responses. It was within this background that we offered Tito therapeutic assistance if the family so desired.

Our work with Tito began in August 1993, when the mother and son duo relocated to Mysore, India. Along with daily one-on-one sessions for an hour with me, he received additional help from the students posted in the AIISH therapy clinic on a daily basis. Tito was then profiled on the Autistic Behaviour Composite Checklist and Profile (ABCCP) (Riley, 1984) and was found to have poor attention, marked hyperactivity, self-stimulatory, stereotypic movements, lack of eye contact, strong food preferences, preference for experiencing sensory stimuli through atypical modalities, and difficulty in initiating motor movements, particularly in the oral area. He also failed to use simple gestures and to initiate any social interactions with communicative intent with another person. There was also failure to exhibit patterns of vocalization in terms of varied intonational patterns, and lack of response to sounds by vocalizing. These behaviors are present in typically developing children between the ages of 12 and 18 months.

Tito's difficulty in initiating oral motor movements was coupled with difficulties with chewing, sucking, gargling, and spitting. He had to be fed and was clumsy while eating. In addition, he seemed to depend on his mother for most of his daily activities, including putting on his shoes and socks and brushing his teeth. We then administered the Screening Test for Developmental Apraxia of Speech (Dabul, 1986), which consists of a series of subtests on voluntary production of speech sounds at different levels of complexity. He obtained a total weighted score of 0, suggesting the presence of developmental apraxia of speech. While the very existence of a condition such as developmental apraxia of speech is debated by some in the field (particularly the behaviorists), those of us who have worked with adults in neurological setups are sufficiently convinced that such a condition indeed exists.

Nevertheless, most Speech-Language Pathologists (SLPs) would reserve the term for a child with some amount of speech, the clarity of which is poor, with no clear underlying cause and no apparent motor weakness that would justify the same. Children with this motor speech disorder have difficulty in praxis or planning and producing the precise series of movements of the articulators that are necessary for intelligible speech. They often present a wide gap between their receptive language skills, or understanding of language, and their expressive language skills or speech, which is absent or highly unclear. Typically, these children's receptive skills are superior to their expressive skills. Seldom would the term be applied to one who is totally nonverbal such as Tito was, during those days. Yet such a total inability to produce voice voluntarily is often clearly seen in adult apraxia subsequent to strokes and other neurological disorders, and I had indeed witnessed the same during my earlier tenure at NIMHANS. It was therefore clear to me that Tito had a severe verbal apraxia, so severe that it included phonatory apraxia with an inability to produce 'voice on demand.' How else would one account for his 'search for his voice' (Mukhopadhyay, 2000 p. 52) while his spontaneous vocalizations, particularly when he had a tantrum, could be heard from one building to the next?

Traditionally, in the practice of speech-language therapy, treatment for developmental verbal dyspraxia has been intensive drilling in speech sound production. I was, however, initially wary of using this rigorous drilling procedure with Tito because of his reservation against 'treatments' and the monotony of speech drilling, given his overall capabilities and sensitivities. I was afraid that it would be counterproductive. Once he had settled into a routine, and with his consent, we put in a therapy program that emphasized motor drilling and speech motor skills. In addition, we base-lined his capabilities in terms of other fine-motor functions by assessing him on the Quick Neurological Screening Test (QNST) (Mutti, Sterling, & Spalding, 1978). All the fine-motor coordination tasks that he failed to do were taken as therapy goals. These included tapping given patterns, clapping given patterns, palm form recognition, thumb and finger circle, rapidly reversing repetitive hand movements, tandem walk, standing on one leg, skipping, closing of eyes on command, and while standing, walking backward, jumping across distances of one to three feet, jumping from heights one to three feet, running rapidly up and down staircases with steps of differing heights, kicking objects placed at different heights, and climbing spiral staircases. By April 1996, Tito had achieved success on all of these except the spiral staircase, which he feared the most.

It was consistently clinically difficult to reconcile this very vocal, but nonverbal, child with the more than lucid thoughts and responses that were obtained through pointing with the letter board. Over a period of time, he used facilitated communication with several student therapists who worked with him, in addition to his mother. However, we never succeeded in using it between us. During his one-on-one sessions with me, my own attempts were geared toward getting a better understanding of the working of his mind, along with probing the nature of his difficulties and attempts at reducing them, often with his mother or a student therapist as his facilitator. Much later, Oliver Sacks (2003) wrote, "Tito Rajrishi Mukhophadhyay (TRM), a gifted autistic child from India, has attracted considerable attention among the general public and professionals and parents concerned with autism." TRM's unique attraction **was his ability to communicate about his autism, thereby forcing us 'to reconsider the condition of the deeply autistic.'**

One of my lasting impressions of these times was of having to deal with a child, adolescent and adult all-in-one, for Tito's responses physically were that of a child, emotionally that of an adolescent, and intellectually that of an adult. It was during these sessions that we worked through issues such as his hatred for the word 'autism,' his reluctance at being tested, and his distrust of the medical professionals. Our discussions centered around his own difficulties as well as characteristic features of autism documented in the literature, such as the avoidance of eye contact and the need to flap, among others. What emerged was a range of difficulties/differences both in processing information through the various sensory modalities, either in isolation or in combination, as well as difficulties/differences in executing motor functions, especially when required to do so.

More importantly, it was during these sessions that Tito became aware **that the rest of us perceived and experienced the world differently than he did.** While we now increasingly recognize that the child with ASD is 'out of sync' when compared to other children in relation to the external world, what we have not paid enough attention to is not only how this affects the child in terms of his day-to-day interactions with others, but also how the child himself has no way of knowing this. Additionally, he has to meet the expectations of adults around him who presume that he experiences the world the way they do. Meeting these expectations and growing up within the framework of not understanding the complexity of the underlying issues on both sides (child and adult), would be enormously baffling, to say the least. For instance, Tito often 'saw' visual images of people and objects that were not physically present, yet at the same time had difficulty in focusing on and accurately locating people and objects that were present in a given physical environment. Similarly he complained that while listening to speech, he had to concentrate hard, as the words sounded like a series of speech sounds rather than unitary words—a similar phenomena that is increasingly being scientifically documented in children with other developmental disorders such as Specific Language Impairment (SLI) and other Language Learning Disabilities (LLD). Paradoxically, as per our observation and for all practical purposes, he was processing speech in real time, like the rest of us. These are but a few examples of several problems we tried to work through. As Tito and I explored these differences in sensory, perceptual, body image, and motor executive difficulties, it was my familiarity with the adult neurobehavioral literature and my clinical experience of working with adults with neurobehavioral and neurogenic communication difficulties that I drew upon in order to enable Tito to resolve his difficulties. Tito continued his therapy at AIISH until November 1996, where the student clinicians worked on increasing his loudness, lengthening of vowels and facilitation of accurate production of individual phonemes, in order to improve his spontaneous speech and his confidence in his ability to speak. By this time, Tito sat through 45-minute long sessions without interruptions and cooperated in all the drills. He initiated communication to satisfy his needs, but showed disinterest in communicating with strangers. He had begun to indicate his needs through speech, rather than solely through gestures. However, his speech was still unintelligible because he tended to break the words into syllables. The quality of his speech was monotonic and he often used a soft voice while speaking. At the same time, Tito's keen observations of those around him and his very pertinent remarks were gaining him a reputation of being a 'mind reader.'

Following my relocation to Bangalore in 1996, Tito and his mother also relocated to Bangalore in early 1997, and I continued to work with him at the S. R. Chandrasekhar Institute of Speech & Hearing (SRCISH) in Bangalore. Therapy at SRCISH focused on improving the intelligibility of his speech, and to this end we introduced the 'shadowing technique' of parallel reading, a technique which was initially advocated to help stutterers gain fluency, but which I had adapted for use with adult apraxics with some success. The technique helped Tito to read better (Mukhopadhyay, 2000, p. 75). Concurrently, we made efforts at increasing his independence and socialization. Given that we did not have access to speech therapy assistants, volunteers from among the students of SRCISH, spent time during the weekends in extending his social activities in the form of attending an occasional movie or spending social/leisure time in the company of students at SRCISH. At the age of 9 years, Tito wrote his autobiography, narrating his early experiences as an autistic child in India. The British National Autistic Society published Tito's autobiography titled, *Beyond the Silence: My Life, the World and Autism* in 2000. And in 2002, the British Broadcasting Corporation produced and aired a documentary titled, *"Inside Story—Tito's Story."* From the year 2002 onward, Tito became the focus of considerable media attention in the United States.

The insights gained from our work with Tito hold significant implications for the understanding of autism. By 2002, Tito had moved to the United States, and other parents of children with ASD increasingly sought our help in working with their children. The growing numbers of such families, coupled with the results of a survey of facilities for these children in Bangalore (Aluri, 2000; Aluri & Karanth, 2002), were the immediate catalysts for the setting up of the program in November 2000 as a tentative trial project. It was the experience built from the many children that we had worked with earlier, coupled with the insights that were gained during our work with Tito that led to the therapeutic framework for the Communication DEALL program. The more than 2,000 hours of 'one-on-one' sessions that we had with Tito over a period of eight years has culminated in the development of an intensive early intervention program for children with PDD/ASD, and other such developmental disorders. The Communication DEALL program inaugurated by Tito on 1st November 2000, started at SRCISH, Bangalore as an experimental program with 12 children, in the age range of 2 to 5 years, diagnosed as having Autism Spectrum Disorder (ASD). It aimed at integrating children with ASD in regular school with intensive preschool intervention.

The most important lesson that my work with Tito had taught me was the complex nature of ASD, as well as the many underlying processes and differences in processing that affect sensory inputs and execution of motor actions in the everyday life of children with ASD. While there are many programs, such as Sensory Integration for sensory issues and the 'More Than Words' Hanen program for communication development in children with ASD that recognize and offer intervention for specific issues, there are few programs that address the multiple issues that a single child with ASD is faced with in a holistic, cohesive manner. Neither do these programs address and monitor the impact of these issues on the growth of the child in terms of their overall development as compared to their peers.

The growing numbers of families seeking our help for their children, coupled with the results of a survey of facilities for these children in Bangalore, which highlighted the piecemeal and patchwork approach to intervention for children with ASD (Aluri, 2000; Aluri & Karanth, 2002) were the immediate catalysts for setting up of the Communication DEALL program in November 2000, as a tentative trial project. It was the experience built from the many children we had worked with earlier, coupled with the insights that were gained during our work with Tito that led to the therapeutic framework for the Communication DEALL program. Given the progress seen in the first group of children by April 2001, the program was subsequently continued. By 2003, the increasing demand to replicate the program necessitated the documentation of the program in order to replicate it with ease and reliability. The documentation of the program, including assessment and intervention across several developmental areas, from birth to six years of age, was carried out with support from the Tata Trusts of India, from 2005 to 2010.

During the last decade, the Communication DEALL program has been used with several hundred children, with constant updates in order to further enhance its efficacy. A controlled study with 30 children has helped establish its efficacy scientifically, as required by evidence-based practice (Karanth, Shaista, & Srikanth, 2010). A long-term post hoc study of children enrolled in the program at our clinic in Bangalore during the years 2000 to 2009 (Karanth & Saxena-Chandok, 2013) suggested that 76.4% of the children had managed to remain in mainstream schools over this period. Equally important are the many parent testimonies to the benefits of the program (http://www.communicationdeall.com).

As the program became established and began to be replicated elsewhere by our affiliates, many of who, unlike us, worked with a range of children with developmental disabilities, and not just ASD, the usefulness of the program for the broader range of developmental disabilities became obvious. As a result, the profile and the intervention manuals are now being increasingly used to guide and monitor intervention for children with other types of developmental disabilities such as cerebral palsy, global developmental delays/intellectual disability, and hearing impairment, after the necessary basic assessments and interventions (such as a complete audiological assessment and hearing aid fitting for a hearing-impaired child) are in place.

3

Communication DEALL

3.1 The Program

Within the seemingly unending range of interventions advocated for ASD, one of the clearest indicators for long-term benefits in children with ASD has been the importance of Early Intervention (EI). Early intervention is increasingly seen to alter the course of the eventual, long-term outcome for children with ASD. Engaging the child substantially when the developmental skills are more malleable and not as pervasively disrupted, as in later years, is seen to affect their growth curves in a positive manner. The U.S. National Research Council of the National Academies Committee on Educational Interventions for Children with Autism (2001), on the basis of its comprehensive, evidence-based report, recommended that early intervention for children with ASD makes a clinically significant difference for many children in terms of better than expected gains in IQ scores, language, autistic symptoms, future school placements, and several measures of social behavior. The importance of a goal-directed, evidence-based, individualized program that meets the needs of both children with ASD and their families was stressed.

The Communication DEALL program, initiated by the first author in 2000, provides intensive stimulation and training (three hours per day, five days per week, over an academic year) to small groups of preschool children with Autism Spectrum Disorders (ASD) and other developmental disorders, in the areas of sensory motor development, communication, socialization, and behavior, so as to enable them to eventually be mainstreamed into general education classes with typically-developing children. The major focus of the training module is sensory-motor development and communication, along with cognitive, social, emotional aspects of the child's development. The specific details of the implementation of this model have been designed to consider the prevailing difficulties in accessing much needed multiple services such as physical therapy, occupational therapy, speech and language therapy, and behavioral and educational interventions, on a regular basis in a holistic, cohesive manner by a majority of the children.

3.1.1 Theoretical Framework

A brief outline of the theoretical framework within which the Communication DEALL program was developed, within the larger context of what is scientifically known of ASD, including its causation and the limitations of current knowledge on ASD, is given below. The logo of Communication DEALL evolved from and symbolizes this theoretical framework.

ASD Cause

Despite extensive research conducted on the topic of the cause of ASD, particularly during the last decade, to date, the exact cause of ASD is unknown. However, a consensus among the scientific community is that the cause is biological, most likely neurological, in contrast to the widely held earlier theories of psychological causation. Based on current scientific research, we believe ASD is caused biologically, though the exact biological cause, currently, is not known. It could well be that there may be more than one or a combination of factors. Further, we believe that irrespective of the exact biological cause, children with ASD have atypical neurological development resulting in a range of developmental difficulties. It is likely that these difficulties are exacerbated by environmental factors.

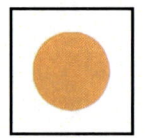

Representation of the core biological cause of ASD

This biological cause, it is postulated, underlies the many sensory perceptual disorders—Auditory, Visual, Tactual, Olfactory, and Kinesthetic that are seen in children with ASD.

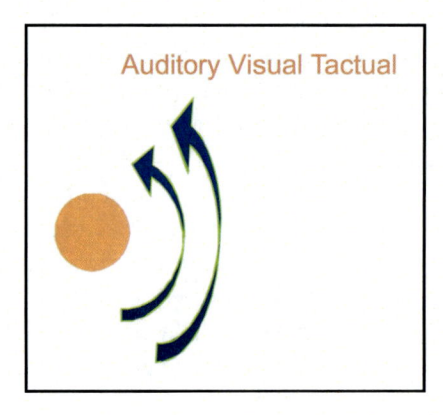

Representations of the sensory perceptual differences in ASD

Theoretically, if one or more senses are dysfunctional or function in an atypical manner in an individual, he or she may develop a distorted perception of the environment. It is our contention/position that, at the core of the difficulties of these children are differences (as compared to peers) in processing environmental input across modalities such as auditory, visual, tactile, olfactory and kinesthetic. The particular sensitivities/ differences in one or more modalities may differ not only from child to child, but also in the same child from time to time. We prefer to describe these as differences rather than deficits as some of these unusual sensitivities are perhaps the underlying basis of the so-called 'savant skills.' Unusual talent in musical perception and appreciation, for instance, can be the consequence of slightly prolonged (by milliseconds) auditory perception. This very same phenomenon could, at the same time, interfere in processing language through the auditory modality in real time, resulting in poor speech reception. Such auditory processing disorders are increasingly being seen as underlying some developmental disorders such as developmental dyslexia, central auditory processing disorders, and specific language impairment, with the borderline between these disorders not clearly drawn. The increasing reports of young autistic individuals such as Krishna Narayan, (2003) and Carly Fleischmann (2012), among others who remained nonverbal during childhood but were able to narrate experiences and memories of childhood accurately, when they did find a mode of communication later, would support the same.

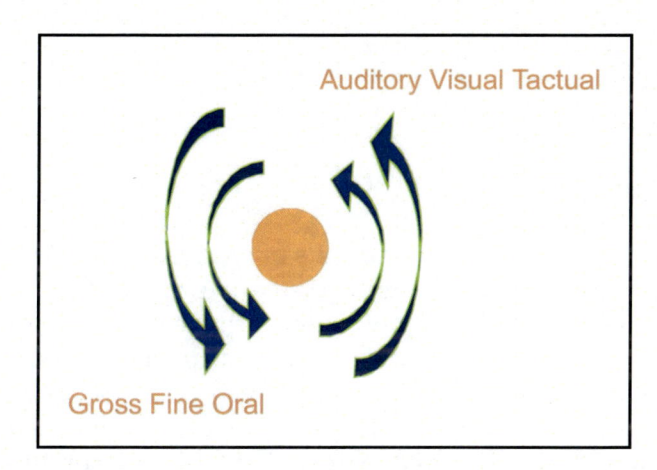

Motor executive difficulties—gross, fine, and oral

While the sensory issues of children with ASD have been observed and documented from the early 1970s, the motor counterpart is only now becoming increasingly recognized and documented. We now know that many children with ASD also have a range of difficulties in imitating and learning motor movements of different types, while some have a few extraordinary motor skills and coordination in activities such as climbing and balancing. Another motor area that has drawn much recent attention is being termed as motor executive dysfunction, which is an umbrella term for difficulties in functions such as planning, working memory, impulse control, inhibition, and shifting set, as well as for the initiation and monitoring of action (Hill, 2004).

Apraxia, or the inability to produce a learned motor movement in response to a command/demand, is well documented in adults with neurogenic disorders. However, while the relatively minor forms of apraxia, such as verbal apraxia, are now beginning to be documented in children, including those with ASD, the more gross forms, such as ideomotor apraxia, or even phonatory apraxia as in Tito's case, are not adequately recognized as of yet. There have been frequent references to children with ASD having difficulties in controlling their vocal volume, often varying between the two extremes of a whisper or a loud voice, without being able to modulate it further, in between these two extremes. The crucial element of the apraxic difficulties is that they are seen particularly when a child is asked to perform on demand. When the same child can and does produce the motor act quite well spontaneously, it further complicates the picture. The impact on learning motor skills, whether they involve the whole body, the fine motor movements, or the even finer oral motor movements required for speech, can be overwhelming for the child (Belmonte, Saxena-Chandhok, Cherian, Muneer, George, & Karanth, 2013).

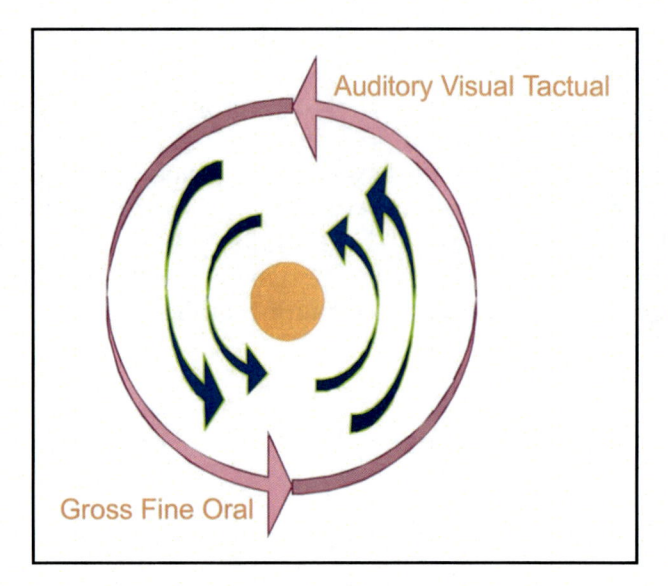

Representation of the issues in communication in ASD

In our model, the communication, social and emotional deficits of children with ASD are seen as consequences of the more basic differences in sensory-motor processing rather than being the core deficits. Subtle auditory processing deficits would not only impact the real-time processing of speech in day-to-day life, but in a growing child in whom the language acquisition process is still underway, would have a greater adverse effect on the language acquisition process itself. At the same time, it is quite likely that the child with ASD does indeed understand the language spoken around him or her, including the specific references to them, despite their difficulties in responding to it in real time. It is thus unfortunate that we often treat a non-speaking child like a non-understanding child, leading to even greater negative impacts on the child. It is likely that the sensory processing issues impact the development of social and emotional skills negatively in a similar manner.

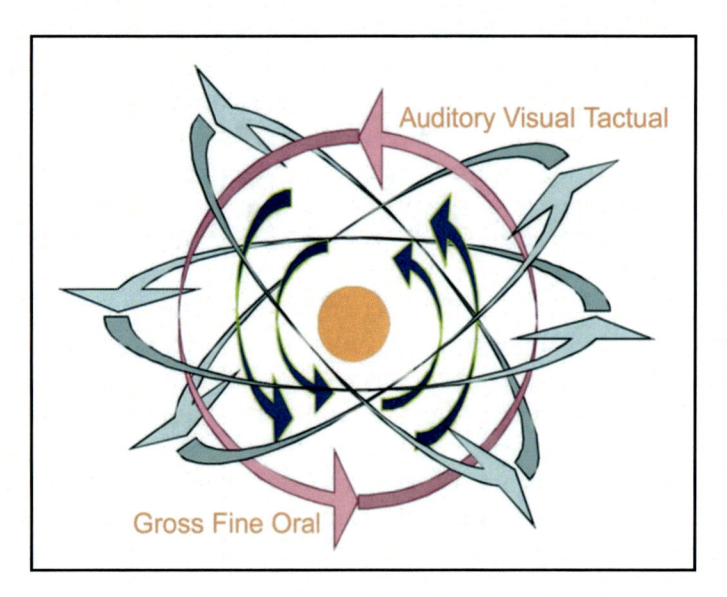

Representation of the behavioral issues seen in ASD

The behavioral issues seen in children with ASD are interpreted in our model as the reaction of the child to the more basic difficulties that he or she is facing and their consequences, resulting in an inability to meet the expectations of those around them and depriving them of the much needed encouragement, support, and nurturing environment that a growing child requires. For instance, the often-observed tendency among children to cling to rigidity in surroundings and daily routines may well be the child's defense or coping strategy to deal with his ever changing, fluctuating world given his or her sensory issues.

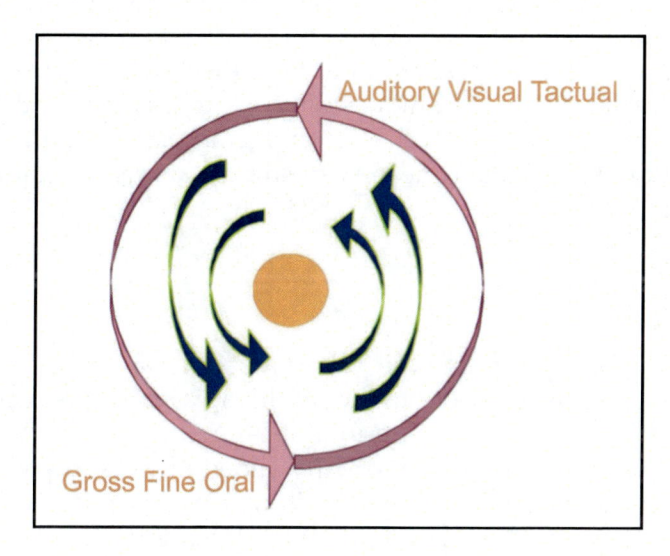

Representation of the Communication DEALL intervention program that targets the sensory perceptual, motor, and communication issues in ASD

In summary, the Communication DEALL program is currently based on a flexibly structured framework of our understanding of ASD. The theoretical underpinnings of the Communication DEALL program are that ASD is caused by a biological, specifically neurological, disorder resulting in a range of sensory perceptual disorders and motor executive difficulties. The communication, social, and cognitive deficits in children with ASD are seen as consequences of the sensory, perceptual, and motor difficulties rather than as core symptoms. In turn, the behavior problems exhibited by these children are seen as their defense mechanism in response to these difficulties rather than being an indispensable part of the disorder. Intervention focused on ameliorating the more basic sensory, motor, and communication difficulties are observed to address and reduce the many behavioral issues.

3.1.2 The Com DEALL Intervention Model

The best practice of Early Intervention (EI) is when children with developmental disorders are identified as early as possible and provided with comprehensive early intervention in order to attain their maximum potential and sustain it over a lifetime. The Communication DEALL program addresses these issues in a two-pronged manner: identify and reduce the issues that interfere with development in a typical trajectory, and compensate and enhance overall development that has been affected due to the former. This is achieved by documenting the issues and difficulties faced by the child, such as the sensory issues or the motor difficulties, and composing a developmental profile that highlights the developmental gaps that are present in each child as compared to a typical peer. These issues and developmental gaps are then addressed by a team of professionals, with the objective of helping the child attain age-appropriate skills in the shortest time possible. Some of the essential characteristics that are emphasized for an EI curriculum are a supportive environment with tasks oriented toward imitation, language, play and social interaction, predictability and routine, functional approach to behavior problems, intensive intervention, family involvement, and planned transition to school. The Communication DEALL program incorporates most of these essential characteristics.

Ideally, enrollment in the program should take place by the age of 2½ years, giving the child the maximum possibility of attaining age-appropriate behavior by the school entry age of 5½ years. Children who attain the goal of age-appropriate skills and behavior by the end of the first or second year are integrated in mainstream school with typically developing peers at such time.

The Communication DEALL intervention program emphasizes the developmental framework using an eclectic approach and specific language-learning strategies. Our intervention methods are not restricted to any one theoretical approach; rather methods from diverse theoretical approaches are applied if found to be useful. For instance, behavioral techniques can and are used by the therapists when needed. Traditional, well-established methods of occupational therapy, speech-language therapy, and education are practiced with modifications as needed to suit the needs of children. Hence, the therapeutic approach is 'eclectic.'

3.1.3 The Team

The teams that deliver the Communication DEALL program typically consist of professionals from several disciplines, such as speech-language pathologists, occupational therapists, developmental educators, and psychologists. With the increasing awareness and identification of physical issues, such as hypotonicity in children diagnosed with ASD, we have recently added physical therapists to our core team. On completion of the medical assessments, diagnosis, and management where appropriate, these teams are involved in the assessment of each child within their domain, followed by team consultation and family counseling. Specific teams of professionals are assigned to groups of children to provide intervention on a daily basis with frequent interdisciplinary consultation, involvement of the family and overall monitoring.

Traditionally both speech-language therapy and occupational therapy are offered on a one-on-one basis in 30 to 45-minute sessions, the frequency of which could vary from 1 to 5 days a week. However, our experience had suggested that while children did improve when they received piecemeal intervention on a one-on-one basis, this progress was not adequate enough to generate the largest possible impact on the child's progress. Even when they make significant progress within therapy sessions on a one-on-one basis with the therapist, the generalization of these skills to other settings, especially with peers in a typical classroom setting, remained poor.

It is a common fact that, even when multiple professionals are involved, the general pattern is that the child moves from one service to the other with very little interaction between the many professionals regarding the management of that child. At Com DEALL, the multidisciplinary team is responsible and works together for the period of an entire year with a specific group of children. This brings the much needed integration in their approach to each child, addressing the range of problems that each child is faced with. The teams provide interventions for the children, working in small group sessions (two children to one therapist), as well as large-group sessions (6–12 children). Children in a subgroup are selected on the basis of the particular skills that need to be targeted for them. As a result, the children in a subgroup for a specific intervention, such as an OT session, may change when they go in for some other intervention, such as speech-language therapy.

3.1.4 Flow of the Program

The overall sequence in intervention is as follows: Once the assessments are completed, the parents are counseled about the child's profile and the intervention program necessary to meet that child's individual needs. The first 6 to 8 weeks target the prerequisite learning skills, along with other basic issues such as toileting and feeding. The prerequisite learning skills include: (i) eye contact, (ii) attention, (iii) sitting tolerance, and (iv) compliance. These skills are addressed first because they provide the necessary foundation for other skills that will be addressed later.

Once the child makes progress in the prerequisite learning skills, the team shifts its attention to the specific issues of the individual child. Profile-based intervention for motor skills and sensory motor issues are worked on with a focus on transfer to Activities of Daily Living (ADL) skills. Language intervention follows the developmental approach with intensive language stimulation within an enriched communicative environment. All possible communication modes including, logographic reading and other visual strategies are encouraged. Individual language diaries are maintained and shared with families. A recurring motto is 'Communication WITH the child not ABOUT the child.' As a child moves toward the age-appropriate skills, generalization and maintenance of communication skills in social interaction and expressing emotions are given greater attention.

It has been our experience that profile-based changes are first seen in the motor skills—gross, fine, and eventually ADL. Then there is improvement in receptive language and cognitive skills. Expressive language skills along with social skills are generally the last to emerge.

Behavioral issues are tackled incidentally during the training, with the reinforcers for the same being uniform across team members who work together in the management of behavioral problems such as perseveration, retention, fear, aggression, ritualistic behavior, and so forth. Structuring events and encouraging the child's anticipation of change are found to be useful in moving the child through the day's activities. For example, when it is time to change activities, the child is prepared by a verbal cue from the therapist. The therapist might say something like, "We are all done playing in the sandbox. Let's put our sand toys away. Now we are going to go inside and eat a snack." This type of verbal cue is very helpful to children in preparing them for transitions in activities. Sudden, unannounced changes are avoided.

Explicitly sharing the reasons for the actions of the adults and what is expected from the child, along with the use of stories for everyday living, and role-playing, help address the many day-to-day difficulties the children face. Preparing for special events, such as eating out in a restaurant, visiting the mall, and participating in a wedding, are often targeted specifically. As children get ready to move out of the program, activities that involve large groups, such as receiving group instruction, and so forth, are focused on to enable the child to function as a part of a larger group, such as those found in a typical classroom.

3.1.5 Time Frame

The question of the time frame within which developmental targets have to be achieved has been a major guiding principle of the Communication DEALL program. In long-term clinical intervention, such as speech-language therapy and occupational therapy, it is an accepted fact that though progress is gradual, it should mirror the rate of growth and progress of typically developing children as closely as possible. Unless we strive to make progress in children with developmental disabilities at least somewhere close to the rate experienced by typically developing children, inclusion will be in principle alone. It is therefore of paramount importance not only to target age-appropriate skills, but achieve them in a given time frame. Only then can mainstreaming and successful inclusion happen by school-entry age.

3.1.6 Assessment

Assessment of children is at best a difficult and time-consuming task. When the children are as young as a few months old and have a range of difficulties, the problem is further compounded. Most assessment tools in the area of Autism Spectrum Disorders are either diagnostic tools such as the Childhood Autism Rating Scales (CARS) (Schopler, Van Bourgondien, Wellman, & Love, 2010) or the Autism Diagnostic Interview (Lord, Rutter, & Le Couteur, 1994) or Autism Diagnostic Observation Schedule (ADO) (Lord, Rutter, DiLavore, Risi, Gotham, & Bishop, 2012) or tools that address particular aspects of the difficulties associated with ASD, such as the Sensory Profile (Dunn, 1999) for assessment of the sensory issues, developed and used by occupational therapists and PLS-5 (Zimmerman et al., 2011) by speech-language therapists. Given our interest in addressing as many of the issues of children with ASD, as well as their developmental skills and gaps, our assessment procedures are also two-pronged.

While the first group of tests addresses the issues known to be affected in children with ASD, the second is a developmental profile that provides a baseline for identifying developmental skills and gaps across several domains. The latter, in addition to serving as a baseline for commencement of intervention, also serves as a framework for monitoring progress over specific time frames. Assessments of the developmental profiles of very young children are generally carried out through checklists administered to caregivers, given that young infants are not very amenable to behavioral testing. This is also true of 'difficult to test' children such as those with ASD. Checklists have therefore become the most widely used tools to identify the presence of a developmental delay and also to provide a basic understanding of the developmental skills of a given child in one or more areas. Checklists are designed by clinicians to target specific areas such as motor development and communication skills.

The Communication DEALL Developmental Checklists developed by us (Karanth, 2007), serve as the core developmental tool for the program and provide a developmental profile of each child. These checklists, along with details of the manner in which they were developed are given in Section 4.2. The checklists can be used for a wide range of children with developmental disabilities.

3.1.7 Intervention

As with the assessment, intervention in the Communication DEALL program is also broadly two-pronged, addressing both the specific issues that are known to be affected in children with ASD, such as the sensory, motor, and behavioral issues as well as the developmental skills that are affected as a result. In intervention, the multidisciplinary team of Communication DEALL addresses specific prerequisite learning skills such as improving eye contact, enhancing attention (including joint attention) and compliance, supporting feeding and toilet training, and reducing behavioral issues along with developmental skill building. Sensory-motor issues of each child are assessed and addressed independently as well as during the process of overall skill building.

The intervention plans are drawn for each child based on his or her profile. Intervention is provided both on an individual basis as well as in groups in order to help the child to generalize and sustain the effects of therapy in peer-group interactions. If she or he is to eventually succeed in mainstream society, generalization of skills learned in therapy is critical. These intervention procedures and the manner in which they may be implemented form the substance of the many manuals of the Communication DEALL program.

3.2 Com DEALL Manuals

In order to serve the requirement of an ever-increasing number of children with developmental disabilities, and also address the shortage of trained professionals, especially in small towns and the rural areas, we set out to document our program in several manuals so that our approach can be used by professionals and parents. These include the following manuals that are now presented here with additional editing to suit an international audience.

1. Comprehensive Intervention for Children with Developmental Delays: Program Manual and Checklists
2. Intervention Manual for Prerequisite Learning Skills: Practical Strategies
3. Intervention for Toddlers with Gross and Fine Motor Delays: Practical Strategies
4. Intervention for Toddlers with Communication Delays: Practical Strategies
5. Intervention for Toddlers with Cognitive, Social, and Emotional Delays: Practical Strategies
6. Intervention for Toddlers using Augmentative and Alternative Communication: Practical Strategies
7. Intervention for Preschoolers with Gross and Fine Motor Delays: Practical Strategies
8. Intervention for Preschoolers with Communication Delays: Practical Strategies
9. Intervention for Preschoolers with Cognitive, Social, and Emotional Delays: Practical Strategies
10. Intervention for Preschoolers using Augmentative and Alternative Communication: Practical Strategies

Ideally, the program should be delivered for each child by a multidisciplinary team of interventionists with the necessary professional training. However, where this is not possible, it is recommended that parents and other caregivers follow the step-by-step procedures that have been listed in the manuals, under the supervision and guidance of trained professionals. The Com DEALL manuals target skill building in each child across the domains of motor skills (gross, fine, and activities of daily living), communication (receptive and expressive language as well as Alternative and Augmentative Communication) and cognitive, social, and emotional development, from birth to 6 years of age. Lesson plans for each of many skills, from birth to 6 years of age are described with clear targets, materials required and simple instructions, along with illustrations. These lessons are arranged in a hierarchical manner which target building the skills of children from birth to 60 months of age. The professional/parent/caregiver is required to begin at the lowest level/baseline at which the child is performing consistently in each subdomain, and train the child in the remaining skills (up to his chronological age) in a stepwise, sequenced manner. When a child remains nonverbal, it is recommended that methods of alternative and augmentative communication be introduced, as described in the AAC manuals, in a similar stepwise, hierarchical manner.

The Communication DEALL Developmental Checklists

4.1 Executive Summary

4.1.1 Background

As stated earlier, there are a multitude of tests and assessment procedures used for children with ASD. The choice of tool is generally dependent on the specific purpose and professional background of the assessor. As our understanding of ASD grows, the lists of assessment tools also evolve. Further, because this developmental program is now being used for a wider range of children with developmental disabilities than the children with ASD that it was initially designed for, it is important to ensure that all other necessary procedures for complete assessment and fitting of aids and appliances, as for example, in the case of children with hearing impairment or cerebral palsy, be carried out prior to developmental intervention.

The Communication DEALL program profiles children on various aspects of development that are relevant for children with ASD and other communication disorders. These include receptive and expressive language, gross, and fine motor skills, activities of daily living, cognitive/academic skills, and social and emotional skills that are attained by children from birth to 6 years of age. An extensive review of literature on developmental milestones in early childhood across the developmental domains of motor development, language development, cognitive development, and social-emotional development was carried out by the research team, consisting of speech-language pathologists, psychologists, and occupational therapists in order to arrive at the basis for a criterion-referenced developmental checklist. The comprehensive master checklist, with items collated from various sources such as books, tests, and websites, yielded a total of 1,808 items covering all domains of development. The extended master list was first categorized into eight domains and then into a developmental hierarchy from 0 to 72 months in 12 groups at six-month age intervals. This candidate list resulted in an uneven distribution of a total of 154 to 380 items across the eight domains, which includes Gross Motor Skills, Fine Motor Skills, Activities of Daily Living, Receptive Language, Expressive Language, Cognitive Skills, Social Skills, and Emotional Skills. The items for each age group within domains ranged from a minimum of four to a maximum of 50 items.

The research team then reviewed the candidate list and edited it further by discarding items that lacked clarity, were not sufficiently concrete for inclusion, were repetitive or overlapped across domains, and were not culturally neutral. This resulted in a list with a total of 945 items with the distribution across domains varying from 84 to 209. The checklist was then refined further with the aid of the clinicians, who were regularly involved in clinical evaluation of children with developmental disabilities and had considerable experience in the administration of checklists in order to verify their suitability for clinical purposes. On the basis of the feedback received, the items within domains were edited/revised further and sequenced in a logical and functional hierarchy to ensure equal distribution of items across the age groups, to the extent possible. The eight to ten most suitable items were retained for each age group on the basis of simplicity, clarity of statement, cultural neutrality, and age appropriateness. This initial review of the checklist resulted in eight checklists for the eight domains with the total number of items in each domain, ranging from 111 to 120 resulting in fewer than 10 items for a few age groups in some domains. In addition, a cover sheet for recording the demographic details of the subjects was compiled.

The research assistants then carried out a pilot administration of the checklist on 60 children who were representative of our final sample, as training for the administration of the checklist and in order to foresee and prevent glitches in administration of the checklist. The results of this pilot were collated and discussed with the statistician, leading to some minor modifications, including deletion of a further 12 items, bringing the total down to 933 items.

In view of the fact that the majority of the children seeking our services come from the urban, middle class homes, with literate parents, the norms were established on a similar sample. Consultations were also held with the statistician regarding the sample size for the pilot and main study. Based on his recommendations, it was decided to have an overall sample size of 360 children with 30 each (15 male and 15 female) at 6-month age intervals, within the overall age range of 0 to 72 months. It was ensured that all 360 children were reported to have a typical birth and developmental history and no significant medical history. Children with significant family history, including a history of late talkers in the family, were excluded. The subjects for this normative sample came from a middle class background. Data collection on the tentative checklists was carried out at the pediatric units of a few local hospitals and a few preschools in Bangalore, India.

In the first phase of data collection, 120 children who were representative of the larger sample, with 10 children in each age group, were evaluated. A review of the data confirmed the essential soundness of the checklist both developmentally within a category and across categories. As per the recommendation of the statistician, data collection was then completed on a total of 360 children between the ages of 0 to 72 months, with 30 children each, in 12 groups at six-month intervals. In actuality, data was collected on a total of 409 subjects of which 49 data sheets had to be discarded since they were either incomplete or found to be invalid according to our subject-selection criteria. Information on nearly all of the subjects was provided by the parent/caregivers. Overall, the parents/caregivers were cooperative about being interviewed, although several complained about the length of the checklist.

4.1.2 Statistical Background

Subject details, statistical analysis and item reduction: The data on the 360 subjects, including both demographic data and the scores on the checklists, were then entered into a spreadsheet for statistical analysis. Our subject population of children, as planned, was largely urban with no significant medical history. The age and sex distribution of the subjects is given in Table 1.

Table 1. Age and Sex Distribution of Subjects

Age Range	Male	Female	Total
0–6 months	15	16	31
6–12 months	14	14	28
12–18 months	15	15	30
24–30 months	16	17	33
30–36 months	15	14	29
36–42 months	15	15	30
42–48 months	15	15	30
48–54 months	18	15	33
54–60 months	12	15	27
60–66 months	15	15	30
66–72 months	15	14	29
Total	**180**	**180**	**360**

Of the 360 subjects, 185 spent their days at home or were sent to daycare for a part of the day. One hundred twenty-four of the subjects were enrolled in Montessori and other preschools, and the remaining 51 were enrolled in Kindergarten or 1st grade in regular schools. Both parents of most of the children were educated, with the majority being graduates or trained, white-collar professionals such as engineers, doctors, business managers, chartered accountants, scientists, and teachers. Only 39 of the fathers and 29 of the mothers were high school graduates or diploma holders. Of the 360 total subjects, 31.4% lived in an extended family, which included other relatives living in the home (e.g., aunts, uncles, or grandparents), while the remaining lived in nuclear families. The majority of the children were from middle income backgrounds.

The percentage of mastery of each item by the 30 children of that particular age group was calculated and is presented in Table 2. Given the variation of the performance of the children on the different items within each age group, as per the suggestion of the statisticians, the items on which the children scored at and above the median were selected for the reduced list. As seen in Table 2 the items in each category for each age group ranged from 4 to 6. From among these items three each with the highest frequency were selected for the final checklist.

When two items differed only partially (in shades of meaning) as for example items such as 'spontaneously shows affection for familiar playmates' and 'shows pleasure in having and being with friends,' in the social domain; an effort was made to replace them with more clearly differing items, taking care to see that such a replacement was from among the items that scored at or above the median.

Table 2. Item Frequency: Median and Above

Age	Gp	GM	FM	ADL	RL	EL	Cog	Soc	Em
66–72	XII	116	119	118	114	115	114	118	111
		111	118	113	111	112	115	120	120
		112	111	112	117	117	113	113	118
		117	117	115	112	113	119	114	116
		115	113	111	115	116	111	116	117
		112	114	116		116	119	119	
60–66	XI	106	107	102	103	107	107	108	105
		109	102	101	107	105	110	102	101
		104	108	105	105	108	102	107	108
		101	104	103	106	102	103	101	106
		108	106	109	104	110	108		107
		103	101	104	102	109	104		109
54–60	X	97	94	94	97	96	94	91	95
		96	97	98	100	93	97	95	99
		93	99	96	96	94	93	98	100
		94	93	99	99	92	96	93	94
		95		95	93	100	91	94	98
					95	97	92	99	
48–54	IX	85	86	83	85	87	90	84	86
		88	87	84	89	86	83	89	88
		81	90	90	81	82	85	81	85
		86	89	85	83	84	88	86	87
			81	81	82	88	87	83	81
					84	85	84	85	84
42–48	VIII	78	79	75	78	79	75	73	77
		75	72	76	79	71	78	75	74
		76	77	77	77	75	72	72	76
		77	74	72	74	72	71	79	73
		71	73	79	75	77	76	77	72
		72			72	76	74	76	

Table 2. *continued*

Age	Gp	GM	FM	ADL	RL	EL	Cog	Soc	Em
36–42	VII	66	68	61	69	70	65	62	64
		67	61	67	70	62	66	63	69
		64	64	69	65	64	68	70	65
		62	62	66	66	65	63	66	67
			63	65	62	66	61	65	68
				64	61	67	67	67	62
30–36	VI	58	59	52	54	54	53	51	60
		51	57	51	60	52	51	52	52
		57	58	58	52	57	57	55	51
		56	54	57	53	56	55	53	54
		53	55	55	51	60	59	54	55
		59	52	54	55	59	56		56
24–30	V	49	44	45	48	46	43	49	43
		47	41	44	47	50	42	42	44
		43	46	41	45	45	47	43	49
		41	42	48	50	47	48	41	41
		45	47	43	41	42	45	45	48
		44			42	44			
18–24	IV	39	33	39	34	32	35	33	32
		35	35	40	32	33	31	37	33
		31	37	31	40	35	38	31	36
		38	34	33	38	37	32	32	31
		33	32	32	33	36	33	39	34
		32	36		35	39			
12–18	III	27	21	30	27	29	28	25	23
		24	22	23	25	30	22	21	21
		22	27	28	24	28	24	22	25
		23	24	27	23	22	29	26	22
		21		25	22	21	30	27	24
		25							

continues

Table 2. *continued*

Age	Gp	GM	FM	ADL	RL	EL	Cog	Soc	Em
6–12	II	14	14	13	19	13	18	15	16
		17	18	17	13	18	14	16	12
		18	13	11	15	17	13	11	15
		13	12	12	11	19	11	12	13
		11	11	14	12	11	12	13	11
		12		18		16			
0–6	I	9	2	5	5	5	3	4	3
		5	7	6	2	9	8	1	5
		6	10	1	4	4	4	5	2
		1	1	2	1	10	7	2	7
		2	3	7	3	1	6	6	4
						3	1		

By reducing the items following the above criteria, the items for the final checklist with 36 items in each domain and three items at each age level were compiled and these formed the Communication DEALL Developmental Checklists. Inter-rater reliability for the same was established subsequently (Saxena-Chandok, Ram-Kiran, Lawrance, & Karanth, 2011).

For this international edition, a review of the checklist was carried out by experienced clinicians working in the United States and edited by native English-speaking professionals. The resultant checklists for all eight domains, and the format for the composite profile, are given in Section 4.2 This new, international edition of the checklist was administered to a few children with communication disorders of the types that the Communication DEALL program specifically caters to, that is children with a diagnosis of Autism Spectrum Disorder, Specific Language Impairment, Developmental Verbal Dyspraxia, or Global Developmental Delay, as well as children with other developmental disabilities such as Hearing Impairment and Cerebral Palsy. Sample profiles of some of these children are given in Section 5.

4.1.3 Directions for Use

Ideally, the questions in the checklist should be addressed to the mother/primary caregiver of the child and her observation on each of the items, from the lowest item up to the child's chronological age, recorded in each domain. If the interviewee is uncertain of any item it may be best to allow her a few days' time to observe a given behavior and report it subsequently. It is also advisable for the interviewer to cross-check a few of the behaviors across domains personally, in order to establish the reliability of the information provided by the interviewee.

While doing so it must be remembered that children, particularly those with ASD, present their optimum behavior in familiar surroundings and when at ease. It is therefore best to record the parents' observation initially and verify the same in the clinic on subsequent visits. At times, a parent might report that a skill that had been acquired has now been lost, and this needs to be recorded. Also, the performance of children with ASD tends to be affected by both the environment (calm home environment versus a noisy environment such as a mall or market) and the individual/s that they are interacting with (mother/therapist versus peer/stranger). In order to acknowledge these issues and ensure that the ultimate goal of intervention is to enable the child to function age appropriately across all situations, a five-point rating scale was introduced. Assessments on the Communication DEALL Developmental Checklist (CDDC) are rated accordingly and quantified. Such a quantification also provides a measure of the gains that the child has to make in intervention, and enables the team and family to monitor progress across time. More details on scoring are given below in Section 4.1.4

It is important to remember that the profile provides a representation of the child's mastery of skills across domains at the time of profiling. It is NOT an estimate of his or her potential. It is merely an observational summary of the child's performance at the time. This simple user-friendly profile is intended to provide a baseline for intervention that aids in planning subsequent targets in intervention toward enabling the child to perform at levels that are more appropriate for his or her chronological age. It should also not be treated as a diagnostic tool, though experienced clinicians are likely to find patterns of performance that are suggestive of different diagnostic entities. Put differently, the checklist cannot be used to make a formal diagnosis such as ASD, or specific language impairment, or sensory processing disorder and so forth. Formal quantification of a deficit, or a description of a specific disorder, can only be made utilizing more formal evaluations and tools. It has been our experience that starting with the profile as a base for intervention often enables us to carry out more formal evaluations at a later date. Again, the profile provides a starting point or baseline for intervention, which enables careful documentation of a child's progress in each targeted domain.

It must be noted that although the Communication DEALL program targets children with ASD and other specific developmental language disorders, the profile can be used with children having a wide range of developmental disorders, including children with hearing impairment, intellectual challenges and/or neuromuscular challenges such as cerebral palsy. On request from our stakeholders, we have in the recent past enlarged the scope of the program to children with other developmental disabilities. More details are provided in Sections 5 and 7.

4.1.4 Scoring

The *Com DEALL Trust* has worked toward refining the scoring for the Communication DEALL Developmental Checklist (CDDC). This revised scoring enables a clinician to objectively measure a skill. The revised scoring system is described below.

Rating Scale

Use a 5-point rating scale for scoring each skill. The scale is as follows:

0 – Not acquired (although the child may have been given sufficient exposure to try the skill, it has not been learned or acquired).

1 – Acquired but lost (regression of the skill has taken place. The child does not show the skill presently).

2 – Acquired but inconsistently present/emerging (the skill is present at times, but not always or is just beginning to form).

3 – Acquired and consistently present, but only in specific situations (the skill is present, but only in one or two specific situations, and has not been generalized).

4 – Acquired and consistently present across all situations (the skill is generalized and hence present in all situations).

NR – No response from parent/Not known.

Samples of the profiles with the 5-point rating system are given in Section 5.

Scoring the Skills

Assessment must be carried out for each domain separately. For children with near typical skills, the assessment should be carried out within each domain from chronological age downward. However for children with suspected overall developmental issues, skills within each domain must be assessed from bottom to top (lower to higher level skills).

The clinician assessing the child must score each skill on the 5-point rating scale. The response to each skill must be fed into the score sheet, against the same serial number as the question posed, within the domain. Assessment should be stopped at the chronological age of the child. Parental report must be supplemented by clinician observation for a complete understanding of the true skills of the child.

Samples of Scoring

Sample I: Cognitive Skill

Skill assessed: Points to long and short.

Response by observation: Illustration of understanding of 'short' is shown, at times; concept of 'long' is shown only when prompted.

Response by parents: This skill is just being taught at school.

Scoring: This skill will be scored at 2 (since it is an emerging skill).

Sample II: Gross Motor Skill

Skill assessed: Claps hands.

Response by observation: Claps hands only during an imitation of a song with the mother.

Response by parents: Claps hands well.

Scoring: The skill will be scored as 3, since it is seen in specific situations/with specific people only.

Sample III: Communication Skill—Expressive Skill

Skill assessed: Names three pictures.

Response by observation: Does not express him- or herself/say any meaningful words.

Response by parents: He or she used to say words until six months ago, but seems to have lost them now.

Scoring: This skill will be scored as 1, as regression of the skill is reported.

Sample IV: Social Skill

Skill assessed: Interacts with peers using gestures.

Response by observation: Is not interested in interactions with peers.

Response by parents: He stays to himself, does not approach any other children.

Scoring: This skill will be scored at 0, since the skill is not present.

Total and Percentages

For a clear-cut understanding of a child's skill in a given subdomain (e.g., motor skills or cognitive skills), the total, as well as a percentage is calculated. Similarly, calculation of the domain total and percentage gives an understanding of a child's skills across motor, communication or cognitive/social/emotional skills. The overall total and overall percentage will display an objective understanding of the child's overall skills.

Calculation of —

1. (a) Sub-domain total: The total/sum of the scores on the skills in a specific domain, for example, gross motor skills.
   (b) Sub-domain percentage: The sub-domain total must be divided by the maximum possible total and multiplied by 100. The maximum possible total can be calculated by multiplying the number of items within a child's chronological age in a particular column by 4. For example a 2-year-old child has the maximum possible score of $12 \times 4 = 48$.

2. (a) Domain total: The sum total of the scores in all the sub-domains of a specific domain. The 'Motor' domain total will be a sum total of the scores of the gross motor, fine motor and activities of daily living. The 'Communication' domain total will be the sum total of the scores of receptive and expressive skills. Lastly, the sum total of the scores in the cognitive, social and emotional skills, form the domain total for the higher mental functions.
   (b) Domain percentage: In each domain the total must be divided by the maximum possible total of the (whole) domain and multiplied by 100.

3. (a) Overall total: Sum total of all three domain totals.
   (b) Overall percentage: The 'overall total' must be divided by maximum possible total for all the domains and multiplied by 100.

4.1.5 Interpretation

It must be remembered that the Communication DEALL Checklists and Profile are intended to serve as indicators of a given child's functioning across several domains at a given period in time. It is NOT an estimate of his or her potential. The CDDC profile provides families and interventionists an estimate of the child's current abilities and difficulties at a glance, and indicates the steps that she or he needs to master to be on par with peers. Even more importantly, it directs the attention of the family to the number of interventions needed, along with their priority and the intensity of speech/occupational/physical therapy, as well as a tool to monitor progress in development or the lack of it, with or without intervention, over a period of time, For the interventionist, the profile provides an overall picture of the child's areas of strength and difficulties, and could supplement an existing diagnosis or help resolution of a diagnosis when it is tentative or unresolved. It sensitizes the interventionist to the needs of the child, regardless of that therapist's specific domain, enabling interdisciplinary interaction and intervention planning. It provides a baseline at which to begin intervention, plan it in stepwise fashion, monitor progress, and review strategies when needed.

4.2 Checklists

4.2.1 Gross Motor Skills

Age Range	Group	Item No	Items
66–72 months	XII	36	Hangs from horizontal bar bearing own weight on arms.
		35	Stands on one foot with no support and eyes closed.
		34	Picks up objects from ground while running.
60–66 months	XI	33	Rides a bicycle.
		32	Catches a soft ball with one hand.
		31	Climbs up stepladders or steps 10 feet high to the slide.
54–60 months	X	30	Participates in bat and ball games successfully.
		29	Uses legs with good strength and ease.
		28	Walks on a balance beam with support.
48–54 months	IX	27	Hops.
		26	Runs well and is able to change directions while running.
		25	Swings independently.
42–48 months	VIII	24	Moves backward and forward with agility.
		23	Increased skill in ball games—throws, catches, bounces, and kicks with understanding of where the ball is going.
		22	Runs around obstacles.
36–42 months	VII	21	Swings on swing when set in motion.
		20	Goes up stairs and down stairs without support.
		19	Runs and plays active games.
30–36 months	VI	18	Unwraps small objects.
		17	Rolls clay balls.
		16	Performs running and jumping activities confidently.
24–30 months	V	15	Throws a ball overhead.
		14	Tries to catch a large ball.
		13	Jumps off the floor with both feet.

continues

4.2.1 Gross Motor Skills *continued*

Age Range	Group	Item No	Items
18–24 months	IV	12	Runs fairly well.
		11	Walks up and down the stairs with help.
		10	Able to get on chairs without assistance.
12–18 months	III	9	Throws ball forward.
		8	Bends down forward.
		7	Carries, pushes or pulls toys/objects.
6–12 months	II	6	Claps hands.
		5	Bounces when held standing.
		4	Crawls/creeps.
0–6 months	I	3	Raises head and shoulder from a face down position.
		2	Watches own hand.
		1	Eyes follow moving object or person.

4.2.2 Fine Motor Skills

Age Range	Group	Item No	Items
66–72 months	XII	36	Likes to disassemble and reassemble objects/dress and undress dolls.
		35	Colors within lines.
		34	Prints numerals 1 to 5.
60–66 months	XI	33	Can copy small letters. (lowercase letters)
		32	Able to fold a piece of paper in two halves.
		31	Uses fingers and wrist appropriately to write.
54–60 months	X	30	Makes precise marks with crayon confined to small area.
		29	Reaches and grasps in one continuous movement.
		28	Enjoys manipulating play objects that have fine parts.
48–54 months	IX	27	Enjoys art projects such as pasting and stringing beads.
		26	Winds up toy by turning knob.
		25	Begins to copy some capital letters. (upper case letters)
42–48 months	VIII	24	Participates in songs and finger play, both familiar and new ones.
		23	Good control of pencil, which is held like adults.
		22	Manipulates clay materials (rolls balls, snakes, etc.).
36–42 months	VII	21	Opens rotating door handles.
		20	Holds crayon with thumb and finger.
		19	Tries new art media, such as chalk, with eagerness and an exploratory attitude.
30–36 months	VI	18	Rolls, pounds, squeezes, and pulls clay.
		17	Pours liquids with some spills.
		16	Uses one hand consistently in most activities.
24–30 months	V	15	Makes own designs or spontaneous forms in drawing.
		14	Turns one page at a time.
		13	Opens doors.

continues

4.2.2 Fine Motor Skills *continued*

Age Range	Group	Item No	Items
18–24 months	IV	12	Can pick up thread, pins.
		11	Opens cabinets, drawers, and boxes.
		10	Scribbles spontaneously.
12–18 months	III	9	Points to recognized objects.
		8	Picks up crumbs from floor.
		7	Able to hold and manipulate objects with both hands together.
6–12 months	II	6	Bangs objects on table.
		5	Reaches and takes an object placed at a distance.
		4	Attempts to play with tiny objects like bottle lid/piece of paper.
0–6 months	I	3	Clenches immediately when something is placed on medial side of the palm.
		2	Puts everything in mouth.
		1	Clenches fist.

4.2.3 Activities of Daily Living

Age Range	Group	Item No	Items
66–72 months	XII	36	Develops strong food preferences.
		35	Finds correct bathroom in public.
		34	Uses phones.
60–66 months	XI	33	Shows interest in household activities.
		32	Performs simple cleaning.
		31	Cuts soft food.
54–60 months	X	30	Performs routines without assistance.
		29	Combs and brushes hair.
		28	Throws pieces of paper and rubbish into the garbage/wastebasket.
48–54 months	IX	27	Ready to learn table manners.
		26	Pulls zipper up and down with ease.
		25	Begins to be selective about what to wear.
42–48 months	VIII	24	Pours juice from a small pitcher and stops before the juice overflows.
		23	Washes hands independently.
		22	Knows how to use a tissue for blowing nose.
36–42 months	VII	21	Feeds self with little spilling.
		20	Able to use hands to accomplish many self-help tasks.
		19	Wipes nose when reminded.
30–36 months	VI	18	Serves self at table with little spilling.
		17	Insists on doing things independently.
		16	Knows proper place for own things.
24–30 months	V	15	Wipes nose if given a tissue.
		14	Holds a spoon with fingers appropriately.
		13	Pulls pants up with assistance.

continues

4.2.3 Activities of Daily Living *continued*

Age Range	Group	Item No	Items
18–24 months	IV	12	Gives empty dish to adults.
		11	Able to swallow mixed textures.
		10	Uses palm and fingers to fill and eat with spoon.
12–18 months	III	9	Lifts and drinks from cup/drinks from a sipper.
		8	Indicates discomfort over soiled pants verbally or by gesture.
		7	Removes hat
6–12 months	II	6	Swallows with mouth closed.
		5	Holds own bottle.
		4	Eats mashed food.
0–6 months	I	3	Opens and closes mouth in response to food stimulus.
		2	Coordinates sucking, swallowing, and breathing.
		1	Sucks finger when placed between the lips.

4.2.4 Receptive Language

Age Range	Group	Item No	Items
66–72 months	XII	36	Understands TV commercials.
		35	Listens to another speaker if information is new and of interest.
		34	Has an awareness of socially appropriate uses of communication.
60–66 months	XI	33	Understands some jokes, surprises, make-believe/pretend.
		32	Understands time sequences (what happened first, second, third, etc.).
		31	Understands more quantity concepts (whole, half).
54–60 months	X	30	Knows colors such as, pink, brown, for example.
		29	Understands opposites.
		28	Understands sequencing of events.
48–54 months	IX	27	Knows difference between top and bottom.
		26	Understands complex directions, such as, "Point to a dog that is black/sleeping/in the box."
		25	Hears and understands most of what is said at home and in school.
42–48 months	VIII	24	Understands words that relate one idea to another if, why, when.
		23	Understands "now" "soon" and "later."
		22	Understands number and space concepts—more, less, bigger, in, under, behind.
36–42 months	VII	21	Identifies hard/soft.
		20	Understands direction words—responds to directional words such as around, backward, forward.
		19	Understands three-step directions, such as, "Please pick up your book from the floor and put it on the top shelf."
30–36 months	VI	18	Shows interest in the 'how' and 'why' of things.
		17	Understands common adjectives, such as nice, pretty, hot.
		16	Understands prepositions such as 'on,' 'under,' 'front,' behind,' etc.

continues

4.2.4 Receptive Language *continued*

Age Range	Group	Item No	Items
24–30 months	V	15	Can name objects when told their use, for example, "Something that you cut with."
		14	Understands who is being referred to when kinship terms such as grandma, uncle, aunty are used.
		13	Understands the meaning of most common verbs, such as eat, drink, wash, sleep, and so forth.
18–24 months	IV	12	Listens to short rhymes.
		11	Recognizes names of familiar people and objects.
		10	Listens as pictures are named.
12–18 months	III	9	Responds accurately to action commands such as, "sit down" and "stop that."
		8	Selects and brings familiar objects from another room when asked.
		7	Follows simple one-step commands, such as, "Get your toy."
6–12 months	II	6	Understands "no" and "bye bye."
		5	Appears to listen to conversations between others.
		4	Pays some attention to music/songs.
0–6 months	I	3	Comforted by a friendly familiar voice.
		2	Looks at you with interest when you talk to him.
		1	Startle response to sudden loud noises.

4.2.5 Expressive Language

Age Range	Group	Item No	Items
66–72 months	XII	36	Remembers lines of simple poems, repeats full sentences and expressions from others.
		35	Uses social speech. Children talk about other people as well as about themselves.
		34	Remembers lines from television shows and commercials.
60–66 months	XI	33	Uses all speech sounds correctly.
		32	Names three basic shapes.
		31	Names six basic colors.
54–60 months	X	30	Asks meaning of words.
		29	Uses possessive pronouns "his, her."
		28	Responds appropriately to "how often" and "how long" questions.
48–54 months	IX	27	Can control volume of voice for periods of time if reminded.
		26	Likes to tell others about family and experiences.
		25	Learns new vocabulary quickly if related to own experience.
42–48 months	VIII	24	Conjunction "because" emerging.
		23	Reflective pronouns "myself" emerging.
		22	Appropriately answers "what if" questions.
36–42 months	VII	21	Corrects others.
		20	Requests permission.
		19	Answers 6–7 agent/action questions such as, "Why are you running."
30–36 months	VI	18	Answers "who" questions.
		17	Answers "where" questions.
		16	Uses several verb forms—eating, drinking, sleeping, and so forth.

continues

4.2.5 Expressive Language *continued*

Age Range	Group	Item No	Items
24–30 months	V	15	Uses two-word combinations ("Me go," "More milk").
		14	Names 5 pictures.
		13	Asks for help with personal needs, such as "wash hands," "go potty."
18–24 months	IV	12	Says names of toys.
		11	Names 3 pictures.
		10	Uses "no, not."
12–18 months	III	9	Protests when frustrated.
		8	Asks for something by pointing or by using a word.
		7	Chatters continuously while playing.
6–12 months	II	6	Attempts to communicate his/her intentions.
		5	Vocalizes loudly/shouts for attention.
		4	Babbles series of sounds that 'sounds' like speech.
0–6 months	I	3	Makes sucking sounds.
		2	Uses vocal expressions of pleasure when played with.
		1	Shows random vocalization other than crying.

4.2.6 Cognitive Skills

Age Range	Group	Item No	Items
66–72 months	XII	36	Arranges objects in sequence of width and length.
		35	Sight-reads 10 printed words.
		34	Says letters of the alphabet in order.
60–66 months	XI	33	Prints first name.
		32	Counts up to 20 items and tells how many.
		31	Interested in environment, city, shops, and so forth.
54–60 months	X	30	Retells five facts from story heard three times.
		29	Matches symbols/letters and numerals.
		28	Tells what's missing when one object/picture is removed from a group of three.
48–54 months	IX	27	Tells whether objects are heavier/lighter (in weight).
		26	Understands daily routines and sequences, in correct order.
		25	Can recall four or more objects seen in a picture.
42–48 months	VIII	24	Tells which objects go together.
		23	Can count meaningfully to 5 (if you place 5 apples on a table and ask the child to count them, she/he will be able to count those 5 apples).
		22	Can recall a three-step direction such as, "Go find the ball and bring it to me."
36–42 months	VII	21	Points to long and short objects.
		20	Learns through observation and adult explanation.
		19	Enjoys pretend play.
30–36 months	VI	18	Chooses picture books.
		17	Concentrates on activities of choice, such as putting objects into a bottle.
		16	Enjoys floor play with bricks, boxes, and so forth, which can be used imaginatively.

continues

4.2.6 Cognitive Skills *continued*

Age Range	Group	Item No	Items
24–30 months	V	15	Little understanding of the need to wait—including waiting for someone's attention.
		14	Knows where things usually belong.
		13	Plays with water and sand (filling and emptying).
18–24 months	IV	12	Recognizes self in photograph.
		11	Very curious about surroundings but has little understanding of common dangers.
		10	Enjoys picture books and recognizes smaller details.
12–18 months	III	9	Puts a lid on a pot.
		8	Identifies self in mirror.
		7	Reacts to various sensations, such as extremes in temperature and taste, textures.
6–12 months	II	6	Looks for an object he/she watched fall out of sight (such as a spoon that falls under the table).
		5	Explores objects in many different ways (shaking, banging, throwing, dropping, finds functional use of objects).
		4	Plays 2–3 minutes with a single toy.
0–6 months	I	3	Recognizes his/her mother.
		2	Focuses on colorful and moving objects.
		1	Recognizes bottle or breast.

4.2.7 Social Skills

Age Range	Group	Item No	Items
66–72 months	XII	36	Enjoys school.
		35	Enjoys social gatherings.
		34	Knows about giving, receiving, sharing, and playing fairly.
60–66 months	XI	33	Joins conversations at mealtime.
		32	Chooses friends.
		31	Follows requests.
54–60 months	X	30	Engages in socially acceptable behavior in public.
		29	Plays with both boys and girls but prefers the same sex.
		28	Organizes other children and toys for pretend play.
48–54 months	IX	27	Prefers to play with other children, is competitive.
		26	Shows more independence and wants to do things alone.
		25	Develops friendships.
42–48 months	VIII	24	Follows rules in group games led by an adult.
		23	Likes group activities and time with friends.
		22	Uses imaginative play.
36–42 months	VII	21	Spends time watching and observing.
		20	Spontaneously shows affection for familiar playmates.
		19	Plays well with others and responds positively if there are favorable conditions in terms of materials, space, and supervision (less likely to engage in pro-social behavior when any of these elements are lacking).
30–36 months	VI	18	Makes a choice when asked.
		17	Says, "please" and "thank you" when reminded.
		16	Participates in circle games; plays interactive games.
24–30 months	V	15	Enjoys experimenting with adult activity (such as using a telephone).
		14	Plays side by side with other children, while occasionally interacting.
		13	Wants to help and please others.

continues

4.2.7 Social Skills *continued*

Age Range	Group	Item No	Items
18–24 months	IV	12	Begins to be helpful, such as by helping to put things away.
		11	Interacts with peers using gestures.
		10	Engages in parallel play.
12–18 months	III	9	Plays ball cooperatively.
		8	Waves bye-bye.
		7	Plays with other children. Seeks interactions with other children.
6–12 months	II	6	Prefers mother and/or regular caregiver over all others.
		5	Generally friendly.
		4	Holds arms up to be lifted.
0–6 months	I	3	Responds to primary caregiver by smiling.
		2	Pats and pulls at adult facial features (hair, nose, glasses, etc.).
		1	Looks at human faces.

4.2.8 Emotional Skills

Age Range	Group	Item No	Items
66–72 months	XII	36	Begins to cope constructively with various emotional states: rejection, disappointment, failure, frustration, success, excitement.
		35	Sense of safety and belonging is important.
		34	Senses growing up and likes it.
60–66 months	XI	33	Tells exactly how he feels: sick, happy, or miserable.
		32	Can easily show love and affection and this does not embarrass him/her.
		31	Enjoys playing age-appropriate games but tends to be more competitive and wants to win.
54–60 months	X	30	Begins to develop a sense of fairness, such as taking turns, sharing a treat.
		29	Demonstrates growing confidence in a range of abilities.
		28	Has good sense of "mine" and "yours."
48–54 months	IX	27	Increasingly expresses a sense of self in terms of abilities, characteristics, preferences, and actions, for example, "Look at me! I'm building a castle."
		26	Enjoys obedience and thrives on praise.
		25	Learns to develop attitudes concerning right and wrong.
42–48 months	VIII	24	Can identify own feelings.
		23	Likes talking and word games.
		22	Enjoys music.
36–42 months	VII	21	Develops a sense of humor, can laugh at self and others when small accidents happen.
		20	Labels own feelings and those of others based on their facial expression/tone of voice (looks at a picture in a book and says, "She's scared").
		19	Understands, at least on a basic level, that feelings have causes (e.g., says, "Sunny is sad because he can't find his blanket.").

continues

4.2.8 Emotional Skills *continued*

Age Range	Group	Item No	Items
30–36 months	VI	18	Shows sympathy.
		17	Just beginning to have a sense of personal identity and belongings.
		16	Takes pride in achievements (e.g.," I washed my hands by myself, or I did the puzzle myself.").
24–30 months	V	15	Takes pride in clothing.
		14	Recognizes feelings when emotions are labeled by an adult (e.g., teacher says, "I know you feel scared about that" and the child calms a bit).
		13	Increases his or her understanding and use of language related to emotions (e.g., says, "Mummy's happy now.").
18–24 months	IV	12	Demands parents' attention.
		11	Curious about everything.
		10	Shows preferences of likes and dislikes.
12–18 months	III	9	Expresses appropriate emotions.
		8	Shows pleasure when familiar adults are nearby.
		7	Actively seeks comfort in a person or object when distressed.
6–12 months	II	6	Shows anger when toy is taken away.
		5	Laughs at funny faces.
		4	Smiles and laughs at baby games.
0–6 months	I	3	Molds and relaxes body when held, cuddles.
		2	Cries to show discomfort or fatigue.
		1	Most content when near mother/caregiver.

4.3 Alternative and Augmentative Communication

It is well documented that a considerable proportion of children with ASD remain nonverbal, though with early intervention the proportion of verbal to nonverbal children with ASD is getting higher. In the Communication DEALL program too, we have had some children (about 25%) who show considerable difficulty in acquiring speech, despite making substantial gains in other domains, including receptive language. Since the ability to communicate is at the core of the overall wellbeing of the child, when children in the program do not make adequate progress in expressive language, despite overall progress, we introduce Alternate and Augmentative Communication (AAC) to enhance the communication skills of the child (Karanth & Saxena-Chandok, 2011). Two of the intervention manuals (Manuals 5 and 10) are explicitly designed to support AAC for Toddlers and Preschool children.

Finally, it must be noted that the checklist contains items targeted for children below the age of 6 years. However, it can be useful for children with developmental disabilities whose chronological age could be above 6 years, but whose developmental skills are below that of a 6 year old in any one or more domains. It could, therefore, be used to establish intervention baselines and guidelines for stepwise skill building for children with a variety of developmental disorders, as well as help to monitor progress. It is also possible that the patterns of delay across the different domains will provide additional insights into the nature of the underlying disorder.

We are open to receiving any feedback on the utility of the checklist with specific populations of children and suggestions for modification, if any, particularly those pertaining to the content area, comprehensiveness, clarity, applicability to the full range of intended uses, concreteness, parsimony, ease of use, and fairness. This will go a long way in revising the checklists, when needed, in order to more fully achieve the targets for which these checklists were developed.

5

The Profiles

5.1 Normal Development

Age in months	GM	FM	ADL	RL	EL	Cog	Soc	Em
66–72								
60–66								
54–60								
48–54								
42–48								
36–42								
30–36								
24–30								
18–24	4 4 4	4 4 4	4 4 4	4 4 4	4 4 4	4 4 4	4 4 4	4 4 4
12–18	4 4 4	4 4 4	4 3 4	4 4 4	4 4 4	4 4 4	4 4 4	4 4 4
6–12	4 4 4	4 4 4	4 4 4	4 4 4	4 4 4	4 4 4	4 4 4	4 4 4
0–6	4 4 4	4 4 4	4 4 4	4 4 4	4 4 4	4 4 4	4 4 4	4 4 4

A 24-month-old boy with normal development. Note that with the exception of a single skill in Activities of Daily Life in which he scored 3 (indicating that this is a skill which he had acquired but not generalized), all other skills up to his age level had been acquired and used consistently.

5.2 Normal Development

Age in months	GM	FM	ADL	RL	EL	Cog	Soc	Em
66–72								
60–66								
54–60								
48–54								
42–48	4 4 4	4 4 4	4 4 4	4 4 4	4 4 4	4 4 4	4 4 4	4 4 4
36–42	4 4 4	4 4 4	4 4 4	4 4 4	4 4 4	4 4 4	4 4 4	4 4 4
30–36	4 4 4	4 4 4	4 4 4	4 4 4	4 4 4	4 4 4	4 4 4	4 4 4
24–30	4 4 4	4 4 4	4 4 4	4 4 4	4 4 4	4 4 4	4 4 4	4 4 4
18–24	4 4 4	4 4 4	4 4 4	4 4 4	4 4 4	4 4 4	4 4 4	4 4 4
12–18	4 4 4	4 4 4	4 4 4	4 4 4	4 4 4	4 4 4	4 4 4	4 4 4
6–12	4 4 4	4 4 4	4 4 4	4 4 4	4 4 4	4 4 4	4 4 4	4 4 4
0–6	4 4 4	4 4 4	4 4 4	4 4 4	4 4 4	4 4 4	4 4 4	4 4 4

A 40-month-old girl with normal development. All skills up to her age level had been acquired and used consistently.

5.3 Autism Spectrum Disorder

Age in months	GM	FM	ADL	RL	EL	Cog	Soc	Em
66–72								
60–66								
54–60								
48–54								
42–48								
36–42								
30–36								
24–30	0 0 0	4 4 4	0 4 4	0 0 2	0 0 0	0 4 2	3 2 0	0 0 0
18–24	4 4 4	4 4 4	4 4 4	4 3 0	0 0 0	0 2 3	1 0 4	0 3 3
12–18	0 4 4	0 4 4	4 0 4	3 0 0	0 0 0	3 3 2	0 0 0	3 4 4
6–12	2 4 4	4 4 4	4 4 4	4 0 2	2 0 4	4 4 3	4 2 4	4 2 4
0–6	4 4 4	4 4 4	4 4 4	4 2 4	4 4 4	4 4 4	4 4 4	4 4 4

A boy aged 28 months diagnosed with Autism. He had been receiving early intervention for 60 minutes/week from the age of 24 months and intensive ABA services at the time of testing.

5.4 ASD

Age in months	GM	FM	ADL	RL	EL	Cog	Soc	Em
66–72								
60–66	3	4	3	3	4	4	0	2
	0	4	2	0	4	4	0	4
	4	4	3	0	4	3	3	0
54–60	0	3	4	4	0	0	0	2
	4	4	0	3	0	4	0	4
	4	4	4	3	0	3	0	2
48–54	4	4	0	4	4	2	0	0
	4	4	4	0	0	2	3	0
	0	4	4	3	4	3	0	0
42–48	4	4	3	0	0	3	0	0
	2	4	4	0	2	4	0	0
	4	4	4	0	2	2	3	4
36–42	4	4	4	4	0	4	0	3
	4	4	4	0	2	4	3	0
	4	4	4	3	0	4	0	0
30–36	4	4	0	0	2	4	0	0
	4	4	4	4	0	4	0	2
	4	4	4	0	4	4	2	3
24–30	4	4	4	4	4	4	0	4
	4	4	4	4	4	4	2	3
	4	4	4	4	4	4	2	3
18–24	4	4	4	4	4	4	0	4
	4	4	4	4	4	4	0	3
	4	4	4	4	4	4	0	4
12–18	4	4	4	4	4	4	2	3
	4	4	4	4	0	4	4	4
	4	4	4	4	4	4	0	4
6–12	4	4	4	4	4	4	4	4
	4	4	4	4	4	4	4	4
	4	4	4	4	4	4	4	4
0–6	4	4	4	4	4	4	4	4
	4	4	4	4	4	4	4	4
	4	4	4	4	4	4	4	4

A boy aged 66 months diagnosed with Autism at the age of 24 months. He had received early intervention for one year and was attending a private special school from the age of 42 months. His motor skills were near normal. He could communicate his immediate needs verbally, name objects, and repeat words and sentences that he hears or heard before (echolalia). Beyond that his use of language was not functional. He could follow routine two-step commands but struggled with overall auditory comprehension. His reading and math skills were above age level and he had excellent visual memory. He exhibited severe delay in social and emotional skills.

5.5 Sensory Processing Disorder with Apraxia

Age in months	GM	FM	ADL	RL	EL	Cog	Soc	Em
66–72								
60–66	4	0	4	2	2	0	3	0
	0	4	4	2	4	2	3	3
	4	3	4	0	4	4	4	2
54–60	0	2	3	4	0	2	2	2
	4	3	2	2	0	3	0	2
	4	2	4	2	0	0	0	2
48–54	0	4	2	3	0	2	2	2
	3	0	4	2	2	3	3	3
	2	0	4	2	2	2	3	2
42–48	3	2	3	0	0	3	2	0
	2	2	4	3	0	3	4	0
	4	4	4	2	2	3	2	4
36–42	4	4	4	0	0	0	4	0
	4	4	4	3	3	3	4	2
	2	4	4	2	0	2	2	3
30–36	4	4	4	3	3	4	3	2
	4	4	3	4	3	4	4	4
	4	4	4	2	4	3	4	4
24–30	4	2	4	3	4	3	4	4
	4	4	4	3	4	4	4	2
	4	4	4	4	4	4	4	4
18–24	4	4	4	4	4	4	4	4
	4	4	4	4	4	4	4	3
	4	4	4	4	4	4	4	4
12–18	4	4	4	4	4	4	4	4
	4	4	4	4	4	4	4	4
	4	4	4	4	3	4	4	4
6–12	4	4	4	4	4	4	4	4
	4	4	4	4	4	4	4	4
	4	4	4	4	4	4	4	4
0–6	4	4	4	4	4	4	4	4
	4	4	4	4	4	4	4	4
	4	4	4	4	4	4	4	4

A 65-month-old girl with a diagnosis of Sensory Processing Disorder with Apraxia. She was diagnosed at the age of 24 months with PDD and received early intervention for a year. She had attended a special-ed preschool program for one year along with individual private therapy for 18 months. At the age of 54 months, she joined a private preschool with typical children. Her speech onset was at 42 months. Parents reported that she had improved significantly over the past two years. At the time of testing she could communicate her wants and needs verbally, understand and follow routine directions, understand most of what was said at home and school, was tolerant to crowded places, and had improved social skills. However, she struggled to process language, follow commands, and imitate her peer group, in real time.

SECTION 5 • The Profiles 53

5.6 Specific Language Impairment

Age in months	GM	FM	ADL	RL	EL	Cog	Soc	Em
66–72								
60–66								
54–60								
48–54								
42–48								
36–42								
30–36								
24–30	4 4 4	4 4 4	4 4 4	0 4 4	0 3 0	4 4 4	4 4 4	4 0 2
18–24	4 4 4	4 4 4	4 4 4	4 4 4	2 3 2	4 4 4	4 4 4	4 4 4
12–18	4 4 4	4 4 4	4 4 4	4 4 4	0 0 3	4 4 4	4 4 4	4 4 4
6–12	4 4 4	4 4 4	4 4 4	4 4 4	4 4 4	4 4 4	4 4 4	4 4 4
0–6	4 4 4	4 4 4	4 4 4	4 4 4	4 4 4	4 4 4	4 4 4	4 4 4

This profile belongs to a 25-month-old boy with a diagnosis of specific language impairment (SLI). He had been receiving early intervention from the age of 6 months. A late talker with no hearing impairment or any motor or cognitive issue, his difficulty was limited to expressive language.

5.7 Developmental Delay

Age in months	GM	FM	ADL	RL	EL	Cog	Soc	Em
66–72								
60–66								
54–60								
48–54								
42–48								
36–42								
30–36								
24–30	4 4 4	0 4 4	4 4 4	2 0 3	3 4 4	2 4 2	3 3 4	3 0 0
18–24	4 4 4	4 4 4	4 4 4	4 4 4	4 4 4	4 4 4	4 4 4	4 4 4
12–18	4 4 4	4 4 4	4 4 4	4 4 4	4 4 4	4 4 4	4 4 4	4 4 4
6–12	4 4 4	4 4 4	4 4 4	4 4 4	4 4 4	4 4 4	4 4 4	4 4 4
0–6	4 4 4	4 4 4	4 4 4	4 4 4	4 4 4	4 4 4	4 4 4	4 4 4

A boy aged 27 months with a developmental delay. He had received 4 months of early intervention services at the time of this evaluation.

5.8 Cerebral Palsy

Age in months	GM	FM	ADL	RL	EL	Cog	Soc	Em
66–72								
60–66								
54–60								
48–54								
42–48								
36–42								
30–36								
24–30								
18–24								
12–18	0 0 0	0 0 0	0 0 0	0 0 0	0 0 0	0 0 0	0 0 0	0 2 4
6–12	2 0 2	2 3 4	0 2 4	4 4 4	0 2 3	0 0 4	4 4 0	4 0 4
0–6	4 4 4	4 4 4	4 4 4	4 4 4	4 4 4	4 4 4	4 4 4	4 4 4

A 16-month-old girl with a diagnosis of cerebral palsy, who had been receiving early intervention from the age of 1 year. She also had seizures and her overall development was slow. On assessment, she showed a global developmental delay with relative strength in receptive language, social, and emotional skills.

5.9 Profile 9—Monitoring Progress

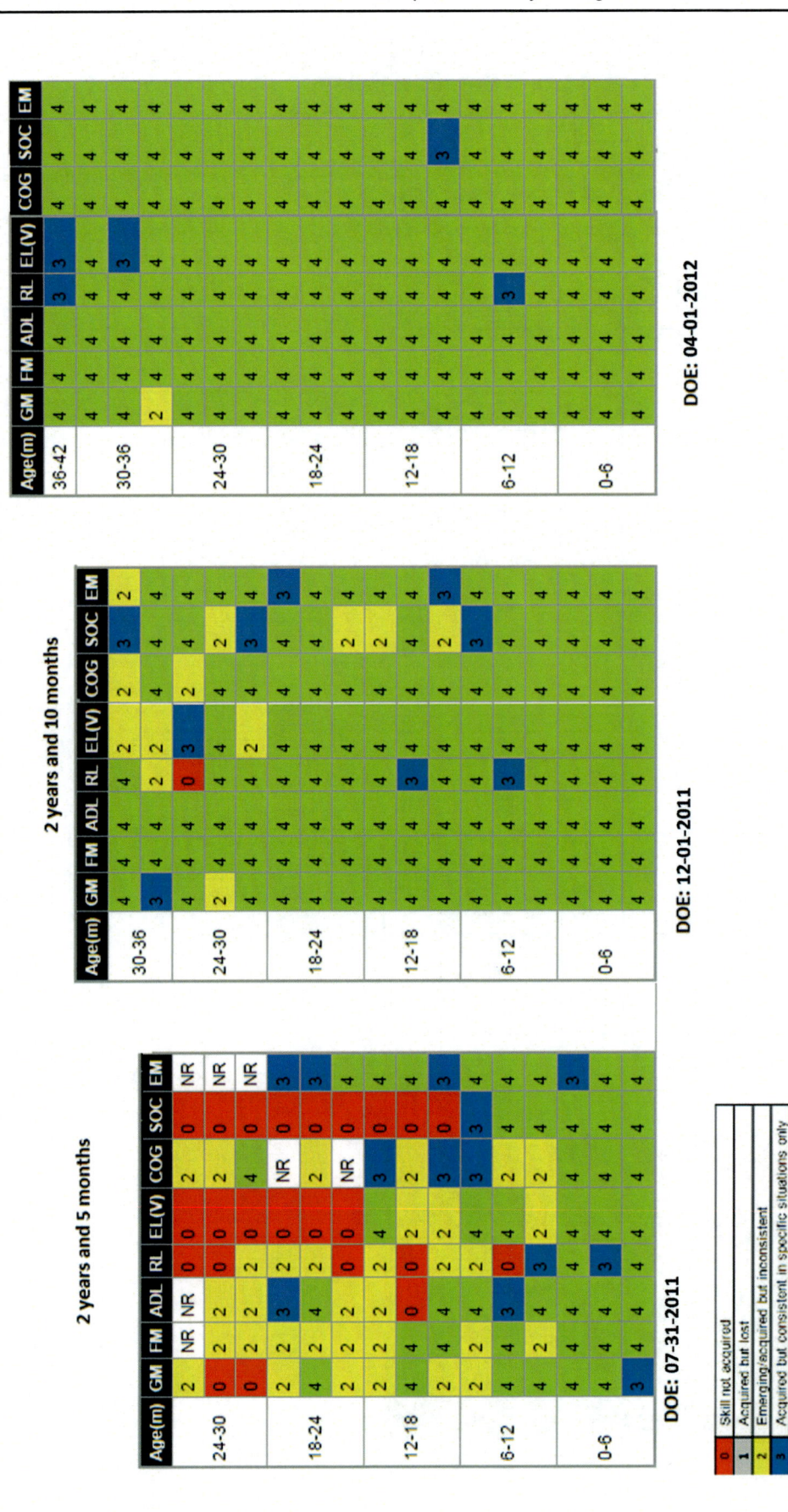

A composite profile of a young boy diagnosed with delayed speech-language development and "at risk for ASD" at the age of 28 months. He had difficulty in eye contact, joint attention, sustained attention, and compliance. He could follow simple commands and point to desired objects. He also had a few sensory issues such as spinning, fear of heights, and aversion to nail cutting and haircuts. He was enrolled in the Communication DEALL program for Toddlers in the year 2011–2012 and the profile illustrates the progress he made across 10 months of intensive group intervention. The child was enrolled in a regular preschool in June 2012.

SECTION 5 • The Profiles 57

5.10 Profile 10—Monitoring Progress

2 years and 9 months
DOE : 06-30-2011

3 years and 2 months
DOE : 12-01-2011

3 years and 6 months
DOE: 04-09-2012

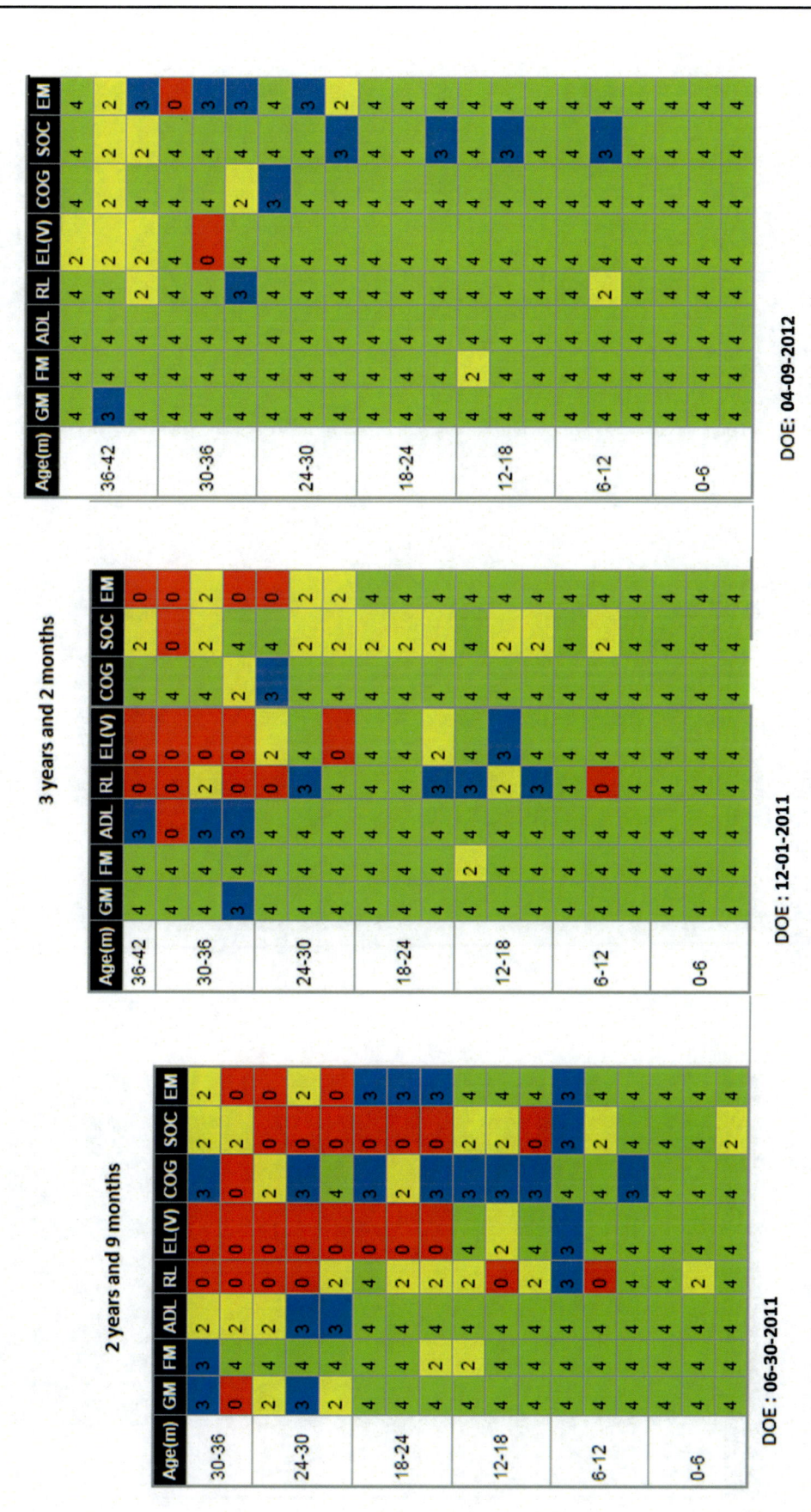

Composite profile of a boy referred by a pediatrician with a diagnosis of being "at risk for ASD" at the age of 28 months in 2011. The child was enrolled in the Communication DEALL early intervention program for toddlers from June 2011 to April 2012 and subsequently in a less intensive small group program from June 2012 to April 2013. The profile illustrates his progress over two years at the end of which he was successfully enrolled in a mainstream school. *continues*

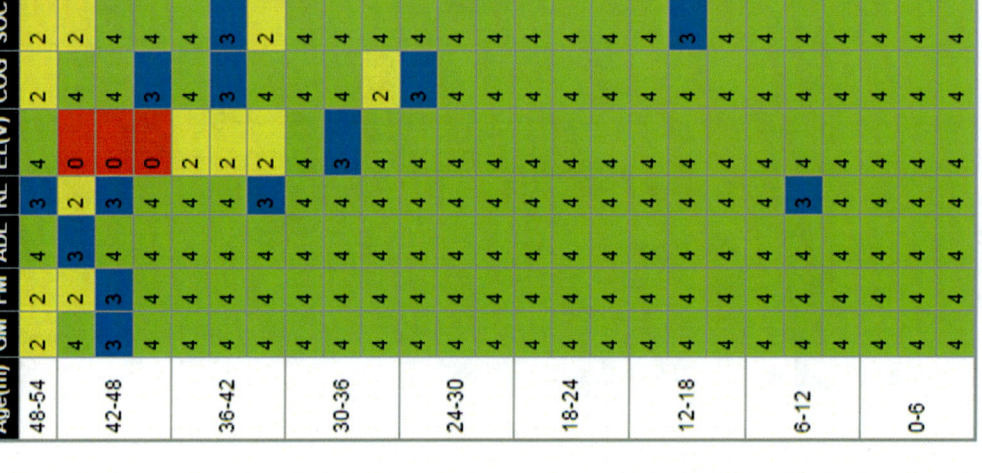

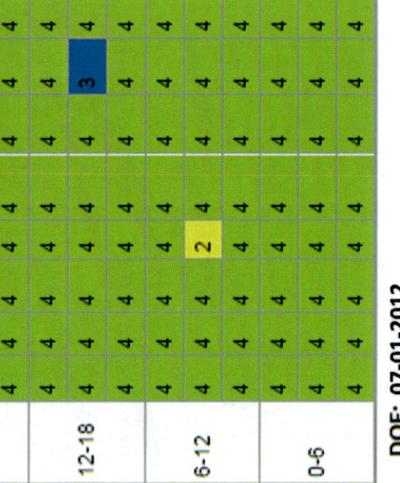

58 Comprehensive Intervention for Children with Developmental Delays: Program Manual and Checklists

Profile 10 continued

Research on the Communication DEALL Program

6.1 Efficacy Study

Karanth, P., Shaista, S., and Srikanth, N. (2010)

Current scientific practices emphasize the need for evidence-based practice (EBP). The Communication DEALL program was evaluated in such an efficacy study during the year 2007–2008. The basic design of the study was a pre- and post-therapy assessment of all subjects enrolled in the program during that year, and on the Com DEALL developmental checklists at the beginning of the academic year in June 2007, and nearing the end of the academic year in February–March 2008, by an independent investigator who was not involved in the Com DEALL clinical program. In addition, a specific overall measure of severity of autism was carried out by an independent clinical psychologist. The tool for this was the Childhood Autism Rating Scale (CARS) (Schopler, Reichler, DeVellis, & Daly, 1980), which is a widely used instrument for the diagnosis and severity rating of autism. The correlation between the pre- and post-therapy scores on these independent measures was taken as a measure of the efficacy of the program. The results were vetted to measure the significance of overall improvement across specific domains. Parental reports on progress, or the lack of it, across these domains were also included, as were the correlations between the quantitative measures of progress and the qualitative reports of the parents.

The results showed significant improvement in all eight targeted developmental domains, across all age groups, in the entire subject population, and simultaneously, a significant decrease on the CARS scores. The average gain made by the group of children in the Communication DEALL program was 17.27 months during a period of seven to eight months. By and large, the parents agreed with the gains in the areas of motor and communication skills, and reported positive changes in social and emotional skills, but desired more changes in the prerequisite learning skills.

6.2 Long-Term Outcome

Prathibha Karanth & Tanushree Saxena Chandhok (2013)

This study was carried out to measure the impact of Early Intervention (EI) in the Com DEALL model, on children with Autism Spectrum Disorders as measured by inclusion and retention in mainstream schools. In order to do so, we followed up the school/educational status of children with a primary diagnosis of ASD who had been enrolled in our program in Bangalore from 2000 to 2009. Data were collected through a questionnaire covering three specific areas: the families' success in following the recommendation given on completion of the EI program, issues in schooling, and feedback on the EI program. The contact modes included e-mail, postal mail, telephone interviews, and face-to-face interviews. In total, 102 of the 296 families responded to the questionnaire. The responses were analyzed to identify the number of families who had completed the program and were able to follow through with the recommendation given on completion of the EI program, any difficulties faced, and family feedback on the program and the additional help that they would have liked to receive. The reasons for failure to comply with the recommendations were also analyzed. Of the 102 children whose families responded, seven had dropped out midway through the program, and 10 had discontinued after one year. Of the remaining 85 who completed the program, 71 were advised to mainstream their children (83.5%) and 14 were advised to enroll their children in a special school (16.5%). Sixty-five of the 71 children who were advised to enroll in the mainstream were in regular schools at the time. In conclusion, 76.5% of the children who completed the EI program were integrated in regular schools, two to seven years after having completed the program.

6.3 Prerequisite Learning Skills

Prathibha Karanth & S. Archana. (2013)

The stabilization of the prerequisite learning skills is addressed early in the Com DEALL program and is crucial for acquiring most other skills. However, literature that quantifies these prerequisite skills in neurologically typical (NT) children is scant. Both clinicians and parents of children enrolled in the Communication DEALL program found this to be a challenge. We therefore took up a study to quantify prerequisite learning skills, such as joint attention, sustained attention, eye contact, eye gaze, sitting tolerance, and compliance in NT children between the ages of 1 to 3 years, in order to target the same in children with ASD. Data obtained on 22 typically developing toddlers in the age range of 12 months to 36 months on these pre requisite skills (Archana, 2009) was compared with four toddlers diagnosed as being at risk for ASD. Children with ASD showed a marked difference in all six prerequisite learning skills in both age groups (12 to 24 months and 24 to 36 months) as compared with the typically developing children. In comparison with the typical children, the children with ASD participated in fewer activities involving joint attention, sought attention less frequently, and sustained it for briefer durations. They used fewer verbal or gestural signals to draw the adult's attention to an event or to obtain an object. While the typical developing child brought objects (toys) over to show an adult, children with ASD did not. The children with ASD also made eye contact with the mother less frequently and sustained it for briefer durations. Whereas typical developing children looked across to see what the adult was pointing at, the children with ASD did not, nor did they point to desired objects. Sitting tolerance was also poorer in children with ASD, and consequently the attending time for activities in one place was far lower for the children with ASD. The children with ASD showed greater numbers and duration of pauses in attention. The number of activities the children with ASD cooperated on and completed was far lower than for the typical developing children.

6.4 Oral Motor/Motor Issues

Oral motor deficits in speech-impaired children with autism (Belmonte, Saxena-Chandhok, Cherian, Muneer, George, & Karanth, 2013).

It is well documented that a substantial proportion of children diagnosed with ASD (60:40 or more recently 70:30) remain nonverbal. In the Com DEALL program, over the years, we had observed/documented that as the pre-receptive language skills improved, gains in overall skills, particularly receptive language, started emerging, with expressive language skills following closely behind. However, in a subsection of the children, expressive language gains lagged considerably behind the receptive language skills. Absence of communicative speech in autism has been presumed to reflect a fundamental deficit in the use of language. However, in this subpopulation, we were inclined to believe that these may instead stem from motor and oral motor issues. The disparity between receptive versus expressive speech/language abilities reinforces this hypothesis.

In a cohort of 31 children, gross and fine motor skills and activities of daily living, as well as receptive and expressive speech, were assessed at intake, and after six and 10 months of intervention. Oral motor skills were evaluated separately within the first five months of the child's enrollment in the intervention program and again at 10 months of intervention. In the full sample, oral and other motor skills correlated with receptive and expressive language, both in terms of pre-intervention measures and in terms of learning rates during the intervention. A motor-impaired group comprising one-third of the sample was discriminated by an uneven profile of skills with oral motor and expressive language deficits and out of proportion to the receptive language deficit. This group learned language more slowly, and ended intervention lagging in oral motor skills. In individuals incapable of the degree of motor sequencing and timing necessary for speech movements, receptive language may outstrip expressive speech. Our data suggest that autistic motor difficulties could range from more basic skills, such as pointing, to more refined skills, such as articulation, and need to be assessed and addressed across this entire range in each individual. (Belmonte et al., 2016).

In order to help children with motor/oral motor issues communicate better, we designed *Point-Out-Words*, a tablet-based software, in collaboration with autistic clients. The software uses the autistic fascination with parts and details to motivate attention to learning the manual motor and oral motor skills essential for communication. The computer software encourages autistic clients to practice pointing and dragging objects, pointing at sequences of letters on a keyboard, and even speaking the syllables represented by these letters. *Point-Out-Words* can be accessed at http://www.AutismCollaborative.org/PointOutWords/

Update on the Com DEALL Program

7.1 Com DEALL Units

7.1.1 Scaling Up the Com DEALL Model

Communication DEALL, the intensive Early Intervention program of the *Com DEALL Trust*, is now being replicated with formal staff training. Currently, twenty-four Com DEALL units are functioning across India. In addition, the *Com DEALL Trust* can facilitate the installation of Com DEALL units in any geographical location, accompanied by formal training and transfer of skills.

7.1.2 Setting Up of a Com DEALL Unit

Typically, the process of setting up a new Com DEALL unit takes one to three years from the time of expression of interest from a potential affiliate to the formal acknowledgement of the affiliate. The process entails the recruitment of a team of interventionists (which includes SLP, OT, psychologist, physical therapist) by the host institution, and an initial two-week training period of the team by the Com DEALL staff. The unit is then set up and a group of 12 children are enrolled for intervention, as per the Com DEALL criteria. The team gathers the profiles of each of these children, and intervention is begun. A coordinator from Com DEALL carries out troubleshooting and the weekly monitoring of each child's progress. Physical inspections of the unit are carried out approximately once every six months, and the unit is certified as an *Com DEALL Trust* affiliate after all criteria are met.

7.2 New Clinical Programs

7.2.1 The Pre DEALL Program

Over the years, our interactions with the growing number of families seeking Early Intervention (EI) for children with developmental disabilities have sensitized us to the need for developing additional programs to support the children. With an increase in social awareness, children are now being diagnosed as being at risk for ASD even before they complete their second birthday. These very young children need an even more supportive environment than that provided for children above 2 to 3 years of age, leading to the development of the Pre DEALL program, with the involvement of a parent on a regular basis.

7.2.2 FMIP: Family Mediated Intervention (Home Training) Programs

Many families are unable to access EI services on an every day basis for a variety of reasons—lack of access, distance, transport, affordability, and so forth. In order to address their needs, we put together the Family Mediated Intervention Program (FMIP) that provides support from the entire intervention team once every two weeks, but with the families doing the actual intervention. The FMIP program is currently being documented and will be published soon.

The increasing number of children who have been mainstreamed into regular schools following EI in the Com DEALL program has sensitized us to several issues faced by the child during successful mainstreaming. Chief among them are the difficulties in transitioning to the school environment, the greater number of peers to socialize with and the reduction in support from the adults in the classroom. Programs that address these needs are very important and we propose to address some of them in the near future.

References

Aluri, U. (2000). *Rehabilitation facilities in Bangalore*. An unpublished master's dissertation submitted to the University of Bangalore.

Aluri, U. & Karanth, P. (2002). Rehabilitation facilities available for children with autism in Bangalore city—a survey. *Asia pacific Disability Rehabilitation Journal. 13*(2), 115–126.

American Speech-Language-Hearing Association (ASHA). (1994). *36*(11), 55–58.

American Speech-Language-Hearing Association. (1995). *Facilitated communication* [Position Statement]. Available from http://www.asha.org/policy.

Archana, S. (2009). *Prerequisite learning skills—baselines for communication intervention*. Dissertation submitted to the University of Bangalore.

Belmonte, M. K., Saxena-Chandhok, T., Cherian, R., Muneer, R., George, L., & Karanth, P. (2013). Oral motor deficits in speech-impaired children with autism. *Frontiers Integrative Neuroscience*. http://dx.doi.org/10.3389/fnint.2013.00047

Belmonte, M. K., Weisblatt, E. J., Rybicki, A., Cook, B., Langensiepen, C. S., Brown, D., . . . Karanth P. (2016). *Can computer-assisted training of prerequisite motor skills help enable communication in people with autism?: Proceedings of the 2016 International Conference on Interactive Technologies and Games*. Los Alamitos, CA: IEEE Xplore.

Dabul, B. (1986). *Screening test for developmental apraxia of speech*. Pro Ed. USA.

Dunn, W. (1999). *Sensory Profile*. Aspen Publishers/Pearson Publishing

Fleischmann, A. & Fleischmann, C. (2012). *Carly's voice: Breaking through autism* (A touchstone book). New York, NY: Simon & Schuster.

Karanth, P. (2007). *Communication DEALL Developmental Checklists*. Bangalore, India: The Com DEALL Trust.

Karanth, P. (2009). *Children with communication disorders*. New Delhi, India: Orient Blackswan.

Karanth, P., Shaista, S., & Srikanth, N. (2010). Efficacy of Communication DEALL—an indigenous early intervention program for children with autism spectrum disorders. *Indian Journal of Pediatrics, 77*, 957–962.

Karanth, P. & Saxena–Chandhok, T. (2013). Impact of early intervention on children with autism spectrum disorders as measured by inclusion and retention in mainstream schools. *The Indian Journal of Paediatrics, 80*(11), 911–919.

Karanth, P., & Archana, S. (2013). Exploring pre requisite learning skills in young children and their implications for understanding of autistic behavior. In B. R. Kar (Ed.), *Cognition and brain development: converging evidence from various methodologies*. Washington, DC: American Psychological Association.

Karanth, P. & Saxena Chandhok, T. (2011). AAC within the developmental perspective: An early intervention program for children with Autism spectrum disorders. *JRCI, 7*(1 & 2), 78–84.

Lord, C., Rutter, M., & Le Couteur, A. (1994). Autism diagnostic interview—revised: A revised version of a diagnostic interview for caregivers of individuals with possible pervasive developmental disorders. *Journal of Autism and Developmental Disorders, 24*(5), 659–685.

Lord, C., Rutter, M., DiLavore, P. C., Risi, S., Gotham, K., & Bishop, S. L. (2012). *Autism diagnostic observation schedule* (2nd ed.). MHS.

Muhkophadyay, T.R. (2000). *Beyond the silence: My life, the world and autism*. Britain: National Autistic Society.

Muhkophadyay, T.R. (2003). *The mind tree: A miraculous child breaks the silence of autism*. New York, NY: Arcade.

Mutti, M., Sterling, H.M., & Spalding, N.V. (1978). *Quick Neurological Screening Test*. Novato, CA: Academic Therapy.

Narayanan K. (2003). *Wasted talent: Musings of an autistic*. India: Vite Publishing

Educating children with autism: National Research Council report of the committee on educational interventions

for children with autism. (2001). Washington, DC: National Academies Press.

Riley, A.M. (1984). *Autistic behavioral composite checklist and profile.* Communication Skill Builders. USA.

Sacks, O. (2003). Cover page of T. R. Mukhopadhyay. 2003. *The mind tree: A miraculous child breaks the silence of autism.* Arcade Publishing. USA.

Saxena-Chandok, T., Ram-Kiran, P., Lawrance, L., & Karanth, P. (2011). The Communication DEALL Developmental Checklist—inter rater reliability. *Disability, CBR and Inclusive Development, 22*(1) 48–54. http://dx.doi.org/10.5463/DCID.v22i1.9

Schopler, E., Reichler, R. J., DeVellis, R. F., Daly, K. (1980). Toward objective classification of childhood autism: Childhood Autism Rating Scale (CARS). *Journal of Autism Developmental Disorders, 10*(1), 91–103. http://dx.doi.org/10.1007/BF02408436 .PMID 6927682

Schopler, E., Van Bourgondien, M. G., Wellman, J., & Love, S. R. (2010). *Childhood Autism Rating Scale* (2nd ed.) Los Angeles, CA: Western Psychological Services.

Zimmerman, L. I., Steiner, V. G., & Pond, R. E. (2011). *Preschool Language Scales–5* (5th ed.). San Antonio, TX: PsychCorp.

Appendix
CDDC Score Sheets

Communication DEALL Developmental Checklist Record Sheet

Name _____

Address _____

_____

_____

Age _____ Sex _____

Handedness _____

PreSchool ☐   Day Care ☐   School ☐

School District _____

Language spoken at home _____

Language spoken at school _____

Parent Name _____

Phone Number _____

Email _____

Examiner _____

Calculation of student's age

	Year	Month	Day
Test Date			
Birth Date			
Age			

Early Intervention

Received	Yes	No
Duration of Early Intervention		

	Gross Motor	Fine Motor	ADL	Receptive Language	Expressive Langauge	Cognitive	Social	Emotional
Sub Domain %								
Domain Total								
Domain %								
Overall total								
Overall %								
Therapy Recommended								

Copyright © 2017 Plural Publishing, Inc. All rights reserved. Permission to reproduce for clinical use granted.

Communication DEALL Developmental Checklist Scoring, Interpretation and Intervention Manuals

Calculation of -

(a) **Sub-domain total:** The total / sum of the scores of the skills in a specific domain e.g. gross motor skills.

(b) **Sub-domain percentage:** The sub-domain total must be divided by the maximum possible total and multiplied by 100. The maximum possible total can be calculated by multiplying the number of skills in a child's chronological age by 4 e.g. a 2 year old child has the maximum possible score of **12 x 4 = 48.**

(c) **Domain total:** The sum total of the scores in all the sub-domains of a specific domain. The Motor domain total will be a sum total of the scores of the gross motor, fine motor and activities of daily living. The communication domain total will be sum total of the scores of receptive and expressive skills. Lastly, the sum total of the scores in the cognitive, social and emotional skills form the domain total for the higher mental functions.

(d) **Domain percentage:** In each domain the total must be divided by the maximum possible total of the (whole) domain and multiplied by 100.

(e) **Overall total:** Sum total of all three domain totals.

(f) **Overall percentage:** The 'overall total' must be divided by maximum possible total for all the domains and multiplied by 100.

Score	Color code and Interpretation
0	Not Acquired
1	Acquired but lost (regression)
2	Emerging skill
3	Acquired but not generalized
4	Acquired and consistent
NR	No response/Not Known

For more details on how to use the checklist scores and intervention manual, visit www.pluralpublishing.com

www.communicationdeall.com

copyright reserved

Domain	Delay Present		Intervention Manuals Required
Prerequisite Learning Skills	Yes	No	Intervention Manual for Prerequisite Learning Skills: Practical Strategies (Book Number 2)
Gross Motor	Yes	No	Intervention for Toddler with gross & fine motor Delays: Practical strategies (Book Number: 3)
Fine Motor	Yes	No	Intervention for Preschooler with gross & fine motor Delays: Practical strategies (Book Number: 7)
ADL	Yes	No	
Receptive Language	Yes	No	Intervention for Toddler/preschooler with Communication Delays: Practical strategies (Book Number: 4 and 8)
Expressive Language	Yes	No	Intervention for Toddler/preschooler using Augmentative and Alternative Communication: Practical strategies (Book Number: 6 and 10)
Cognitive skill	Yes	No	Intervention for Toddler with Cognitive, Social, Emotional Delays: Practical strategies (Book Number 5)
Social	Yes	No	Intervention for preschooler with Cognitive, Social, Emotional Delays: Practical strategies (Book Number 9)
Emotional	Yes	No	

Copyright © 2017 Plural Publishing, Inc. All rights reserved. Permission to reproduce for clinical use granted.

Communication DEALL Developmental Profile

Name: Sex:

Age: Date:

Age	Group	No:	GM	FM	ADL	RL	EL	Cog	Soc	EM
66-72	XII	36								
		35								
		34								
60-66	XI	33								
		32								
		31								
54-60	X	30								
		29								
		28								
48-54	IX	27								
		26								
		25								
42-48	VIII	24								
		23								
		22								
36-42	VII	21								
		20								
		19								
30-36	VI	18								
		17								
		16								
24-30	V	15								
		14								
		13								
18-24	IV	12								
		11								
		10								
12-18	III	9								
		8								
		7								
6-12	II	6								
		5								
		4								
0-6	I	3								
		2								
		1								
Sub Domain %										
Domain total										
Domain %										
Over all Total						**Over all %**			

Copyright © 2017 Plural Publishing, Inc. All rights reserved. Permission to reproduce for clinical use granted.

Communication DEALL Developmental Checklist Lesson Plan

Domain	Goals	Section Number	Book Number	Page Number
Prerequisite Learning Skills				
Gross Motor Goal				
Fine Motor Goal				
ADL Goal				
Receptive Language Goal				
Expressive Language Goal				
AAC				
Cognitive Goal				
Social Goal				
Emotional Goal				

Copyright © 2017 Plural Publishing, Inc. All rights reserved. Permission to reproduce for clinical use granted.